Wound Care

Edited by

STEPHEN WESTABY
BSc MB BS FRCS

Cardiothoracic Surgeon
Hammersmith Hospital and
Royal Postgraduate Medical School
London

William Heinemann Medical Books Ltd
London

To
My parents and Gemma

First published 1985

ISBN: 0–433–35501–8

Typeset by Inforum Ltd, Portsmouth
Printed in Singapore by Imago

Contents

Acknowledgements

The Editor and publishers particularly wish to thank:
Johnson & Johnson whose generous financial assistance
  has made publication of this book possible and also for
  valuable technical advice.

Acknowledgements are also due to:
The Editor of the *Nursing Times* for permission to reprint
  selected material from their series 'Wound Care'
  (1981/82) and for the loan of film of some of the artwork.
The Editor of *The British Journal of Hospital Medicine* and
  Michael P. Quinlan for permission to reprint Chapter
  17 which appeared in May 1983 under the title 'Eye
  Injury' and for the loan of the film.
Imperial Chemical Industries, Pharmaceuticals Division
  and Edward J. L. Lowbury for permission to reprint
  part of their booklet *Management and Control of Infection in
  Burn Injuries* (1980) as well as the loan of film for
  Chapter 19.

Foreword

The proper management of accidental wounds and surgical incisions, the processes of healing and the complications which result remain basic to surgical practice. In spite of a great deal of research and a voluminous literature these processes, and in particular the factors which adversely affect healing, remain incompletely understood. Gaps remain in our knowledge of the most appropriate forms of treatment, the prevention of infection and the management of wounds afflicting particular parts of the body. Also there are few texts solely devoted to these aspects. This volume has been prepared by a young cardiac surgeon with a broad experience of elective and emergency surgery in an attempt to draw together much of the available knowledge. The aim of the book is to present an up-to-date account of wound care and the approach is essentially practical.

The Editor has drawn together a number of experienced surgeons and other authorities to cover the field, beginning with the fundamentals of the subject including an historical review, and ending with medico-legal considerations.

It is a pleasure to introduce this book and to wish it well in the hope that it will be valuable to practising surgeons, both trainee and consultant, across the span of specialists and to nurses, medical students and others involved in wound care.

Professsor L. H. Blumgart BDS MD FRCS,
Director,
Department of Surgery,
Hammersmith Hospital and Royal Postgraduate Medical School, London.

List of Contributors

MICHAEL BEVERLY, MB BS FRCS
Registrar, Dept of Orthopaedics, Hammersmith Hospital, London.

JOHN W. P. BRADLEY, BM BCh FRCS
Consultant Surgeon, Hillingdon and Mount Vernon Hospitals, Middx.

IAN CAPPERAULD, FRCS
Executive Director, Research and Development, Ethicon Ltd.

J. S. CASON (dec'd), MB ChB FRCS
Late Consultant Surgeon, Birmingham Accident Hospital.

RICHARD COOMBS, MA BM BChir FRCS MRCP
Consultant Orthopaedic Surgeon and Senior Lecturer, Hammersmith Hospital and Royal Postgraduate Medical School, London.

WILLIAM G. EVERETT, MCh MA BM BCh FRCS
Consultant Surgeon, Addenbrooke's Hospital, Cambridge.

WILLIAM S. FOUNTAIN, MB ChB FRCS
Senior Registrar in Cardiothoracic Surgery, Western General Hospital, Edinburgh.

ROBERT D. ILLINGWORTH, MB BS FRCS
Consultant Neurosurgeon, Charing Cross and Middlesex Hospitals, London.

BERNARD KNIGHT, MD MRCP FRCPath DMJPath, Barrister
Professor of Forensic Pathology, University of Wales College of Medicine, Cardiff.

EDWARD J. LOWBURY, MA DM FRCS FRCP FRCPath
Consultant Microbiologist and Pathologist, Birmingham Accident Hospital.

AVERIL O. MANSFIELD, ChM MB ChB FRCS
Consultant Vascular Surgeon, Hammersmith and St Mary's Hospitals; Senior Lecturer, Royal Postgraduate Medical School, London.

A. KEITH MANT, MD FRCP FRCPath DMJPath
Head, Dept of Forensic Medicine, Guy's Hospital; Professor of Forensic Medicine, University of London; Hon Consultant in Forensic Medicine, King's College Hospital; Visiting Lecturer in Medical Jurisprudence and Toxicology, St Mary's Hospital, London.

LT COL MICHAEL OWEN-SMITH, MS FRCS, Lt Col RAMC(V)
Consultant Surgeon, Hinchingbrooke Hospital, Huntingdon, Cambs.

MICHAEL P. QUINLAN, MB ChB DO FRCS
Consultant Ophthalmic Surgeon, Victoria Eye Hospital, Hereford.

ROY SANDERS, BSc MB BS FRCS
Consultant Plastic Surgeon, Mount Vernon, Royal National Orthopaedic and Middlesex Hospitals, London.

ALISON THORN, SRN DipN(Lond)
Senior Sister, Accident and Emergency Dept., Kent and Sussex Hospital, Tunbridge Wells, Kent.

T. D. TURNER, MPharm FPS FLS MCPP
Director, Surgical Dressings Research Unit, Welsh
School of Pharmacy, UWIST, Cardiff.

STEPHEN WESTABY, BSc MB BS FRCS
Cardiothoracic Surgeon, Hammersmith Hospital and
Royal Postgraduate Medical School, London.

SYDNEY WHITE, SRN SCM ONC
Nursing Officer, Infection Control, Tunbridge Wells
Health District, Kent.

Chapter 1

Introduction

Stephen Westaby

During the course of man's evolution he lost a valuable defence mechanism, the ability for total regeneration of a part by pleuripotent cells. This power is retained by certain sea creatures and amphibians such as the newt, but higher animals have lost their regenerative capacity almost completely and accepted in its place a much less complicated but, nevertheless, important process – the phenomenon of healing.

Although the ability to heal is a valuable asset, it can be regarded at best as a method for preserving life and cannot be compared to the more pristine function of regeneration. Moreover, the formation of scar tissue, the characteristic of human repair, can be detrimental even to the point of destroying the organism it seeks to preserve. Consider, for instance, the potentially fatal deformity of heart valve leaflets during healing after rheumatic fever and the development of cirrhosis after hepatitis (Fig 1.1).

We now know that healing proceeds through a series of well ordered cellular and biochemical events and that many factors may influence, both favourably and unfavourably, the manner in which repair proceeds. Persistent trauma to the continuingly fluttering and inflamed heart valve, invasion of pathogenic bacteria in a contaminated laceration, lack of essential chemicals in scurvy or repeated disturbance of a wound, as in a poorly splinted fracture, all adversely affect healing, but can be controlled in various ways.

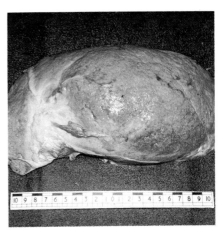

Fig 1.1 Cirhosis of the liver showing that the formation of scar tissue can be detrimental.

Because of the ability to influence the process of healing favourably by attention to detail, a fundamental knowledge of the basic principles of wound healing and care are important in virtually every field of medicine and nursing. Teaching in this field is often limited or confused, however, by fastidious attention to traditional or complicated dressing techniques which are ritualistic and add nothing to the proper care of the patient. In addition, doctors are often slow to discuss current approaches to wound care, perhaps because wounds are usually considered 'surgical property' and most surgeons take wound healing for granted.

It is true that whatever outrage is perpetrated, most wounds in an otherwise healthy person heal quickly, even in the presence of a limited degree of infection. Nowadays wound infection with dehiscence, keloid formation or unsightly scarring are all largely preventable. However, they still occur with unacceptable regularity and account for a considerable amount of patient misery, nursing time and expense.

It is unacceptable to regard complications as inevitable though mistakes still occur despite good intentions. For instance, desiccation of the surface of an open wound hinders the process of epithelisation, yet for many years dry dressings were applied to the surface of fresh wounds. Wounds in the accident department are frequently treated blindly with antibiotics and tetanus toxoid without taking an adequate history or attempting surgically to debride and remove dead, damaged or severely contaminated tissue. Dirty lacerations are often closed primarily with sutures only to return two or three days later with a painful, swollen limb, enlarged and tender lymph glands and the same sutures embedded deeply in inflamed oedematous tissue.

Consequently, it is increasingly apparent that a sound understanding of the treatment of wounds requires not only a knowledge of the mechanism of healing, but also an insight into microbiology and its relevance to the prevention and therapy of wound infection. Nevertheless, the most important consideration is the patient as a whole and we must not forget the patient's own attitude to his wound. The patient with a traumatic wound, rushed to hospital in heavily dramatised circumstances, is always terrified by the prospect ahead of him. The true nature and extent of the injury are often unknown to him at this stage, and a calming influence has initially more therapeutic benefit than pain-killing drugs and antiseptic gauze. This is not superstition; it has a physiological basis in that adrenaline adversely affects wound healing.

Many surgical patients attach a great deal of mystique to their wound. A significant amount of anxiety exists in the patient's mind before and after operation while he passes the time imagining a host of terrible things that might happen if he coughs, breathes deeply, or in any way disturbs the status quo. Although bursting of a wound is a real and frightening thing for patient and nurse alike, it is fortunately very uncommon and generally not at all related to the patient's activities. Yet probably every patient imagines his wound may burst when the sutures are removed, especially when this is done as early as the third day. He, therefore, lies perfectly still and far greater complications such as pneumonia or venous thrombosis may result from immobility.

It is our obligation to consider the patient as a whole and not to be mesmerised by the wound in the same way. Staff should discuss the wound with the patient, determine his 'concepts' of the wound and try to eliminate false ideas that serve no useful purpose and may well prove detrimental. This approach does much to relieve the depression, apathy and physical discomfort of the wounded patient.

THE CLASSIFICATION OF WOUNDS

Many different classifications of wounds have been offered and frankly do not warrant the importance attached to them. Some refer to the anatomical site, others to the depth of the wound and the layers of tissue damaged. From a treatment standpoint there are essentially two types of wounds: those which are characterised by loss of tissue and those in which no tissue has been lost (Figs 1.2; 1.3).

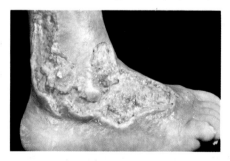

Fig 1.2   A leg ulcer following streptococcal infection; an example of a wound with tissue loss.

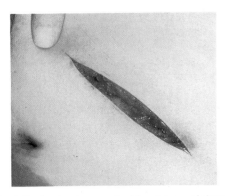

Fig 1.3   Incised wound without loss of tissue.

Cleanly incised lacerations and surgical incisions are examples of wounds without tissue loss and avulsion injuries, burns and varicose ulcers are examples of wounds which, in addition to interruption in surface continuity, result in destruction of tissue. Even surgical (incised) wounds vary greatly in severity from the simple, superficial clean wound, for instance after inguinal herniorrhaphy, to the vastly more serious, deep, bacteriologically contaminated wound during laparotomy in an obese person for perforated diverticular disease with peritonitis. The severity of the wound determines many things such as duration of healing, probability of complications and, from a practical standpoint, the presence of tubes, drains, or suction devices.

The most important question which must be answered for every wound, with or without tissues loss is, can immediate closure be done safely? If the wound can be closed by suturing the edges together or by a graft of some kind, a decision must be made as to whether closure may be immediate (primary closure), or delayed (delayed primary closure) or deferred altogether (healing by secondary intention) (*see* Chap 5). This whole question revolves around the likelihood of bacterial contamination and the risk of infection. To close a wound, with or without tissue loss, by suture or graft, in the presence of bacterial contamination risks disaster and may seriously threaten the life (or the

limb) of the patient. This is because certain virulent bacteria thrive in an atmosphere without oxygen especially in the blood clot, serum or damaged tissue beneath closed skin. As a medical student it was alarming to see extensive, traumatic wounds surgically debrided (and made into larger wounds) and left wide open. One's natural instinct is to cover and repair the defect as soon as possible. However, the consequences of gas gangrene or extensive streptococcal cellulitis after suture of a simple, dirty laceration are certainly more shocking.

In practical and therapeutic terms the most useful classification of wounds does not relate to site, size, or depth of a wound or whether traumatically or surgically created, but to whether the wound is clean or contaminated. Practically all traumatic wounds must be considered bacteriologically contaminated and always if they contain foreign bodies, or dead and devitalised tissue. Clean wounds without tissue loss may be closed safely by tapes or sutures, and clean wounds with tissue loss, for instance after wide excision of a melanoma, may be closed by skin grafts. Contaminated wounds must never be closed immediately without radical removal of all damaged tissue and this may include important structures such as nerve

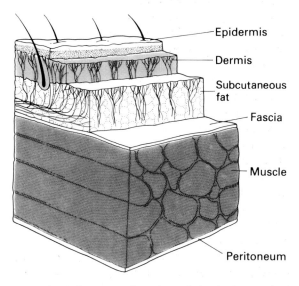

Fig 1.4   Cross-section of an abdominal wound.

or bone in some cases. Even then, most surgeons agree that closure should be delayed for several days until the risks of infection have passed, or indefinitely, when the wound will heal by granulation (secondary intention).

Proper management of any wound, therefore, requires a knowledge of the basic principles of bacteriology and wound healing. Considering a patient after thyroidectomy and another after laparotomy for perforated bowel with peritonitis, why, in the first instance, can tapes or clips be removed on the third day, while, in the second, the wound is not sutured, taped or clipped, but left open and irrigated? In each case the anatomical layers traversed are similar – skin, fat, fascia and muscle (Fig 1.4). Bacterial contamination is part of the story, but not the whole of it.

The aim of this book is to provide those involved in wound care with sound and, more especially, safe principles on which to base their future experience. Experience gained without prior knowledge of the fundamentals of wound care is too often acquired at the expense of the patient. Ambroise Paré said: 'I make the wound and God heals it.' Although this may still apply, we are now in a much better situation to influence this process beneficially.

Chapter 2

The History of Wound Treatment

Bernard Knight

Leaves, feathers, honey, tree bark, rags and paper have all played a part in wound treatment through the ages. Dried goat's dung, honey boiled in vinegar, heads of soldier ants and boiled puppies . . . the list sounds as if it came from Macbeth's witches on the blasted heath. Yet these are but a tiny part of the saga of wound treatment through the ages. It has been a long road from mud dressings to aerosol sprays – a road with many blind alleys and double bends.

We have no way of knowing how earliest man dealt with his wounds, although the availability of simple remedies easily to hand and comparisons with primitive tribes today allow us to make some inspired guesses. Wounds in ancient times were almost all from accidents and warfare, rather than surgically induced, although it must be remembered that as far back as the New Stone Age, the semi-magical operation of skull trephining was carried out.

EVIDENCE

Many of the skulls found by archaeologists have holes which show clear evidence of bone healing, indicating that the patient survived for a considerable time after the operation. Also by analogy with many modern races, ritual circumcision in both sexes was carried out so that the care of surgical wounds was by no means unknown to primitive man.

The mortality rate from all wounds must have been very high, although it has been suggested that two factors might have made this less than we might expect. First, the gross infant and child mortality, probably at least two-thirds, would have selected the fittest for adulthood. In addition, it may well be that with a tiny, sparse population, cross-infection and the development of many pathogens may have

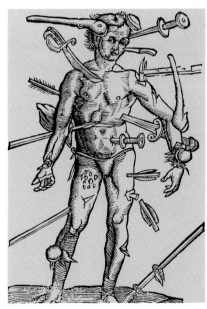

Fig 2.1 The wound man, showing positions for ligation of arteries or for blood letting, 1593. (By courtesy of Ann Ronan Picture Library and E.P. Goldschmidt & Co.)

been considerably less than in our crowded, septic world today.

Most trauma that was not rapidly fatal would have consisted of lacerations and fractures and the first attempts at caring for the victims would be to check bleeding, to try to replace the edges of torn tissues and to cover up the wounds. The urge to haemostasis was instinctive, as blood has always been considered the essence of life itself. Pressure, covering with mud or even sand, as some American Indians do or, in northern climates, covering with snow, may have been used then as now.

INSTINCT

Covering with leaves, bird's feathers and leather are other contemporary primitive methods which may not only have stopped bleeding, but hidden the wound from sight. This was another natural instinct, arising partly from the psychological urge to hide misfortune from view, but also from the widespread belief in many cultures, even until recent times, that exposure to air was bad for a wound.

Although, until the scientific advances of men like Pasteur in the last century, this urge to exclude the air had no logical foundation, it may inadvertently have done much good over the millenia in shielding the damaged tissues from an overload of bacteria – not that keeping air from a laceration packed with fresh cow-dung was likely to make much difference to its sterility!

We know little about methods of suturing wounds until about 4000 years ago, but probably the methods of native people both today and in the recent past must have originated in the dawn of history. Some African tribes use long, curved acacia thorns which are passed through holes in the wound flaps previously punched with a sharp point. A length of vegetable fibre is then wound back and forth between the projecting ends, like winding a clothes line on a cleat, so that the wound edges are drawn together. When the wound is healed, the fibres are removed and the thorns slid out.

No splints have survived from before ancient Egyptian times, although primitive people now use branches and bark to immobilise fractures. The Egyptians used embalming linen stiffened with glue as splints. Some Australian aborigines still encase a broken limb with thick mud and leave it to harden in the sun to make a very effective cast.

SUBSTANCES

A whole volume could be written on the many substances used as wound dressings through

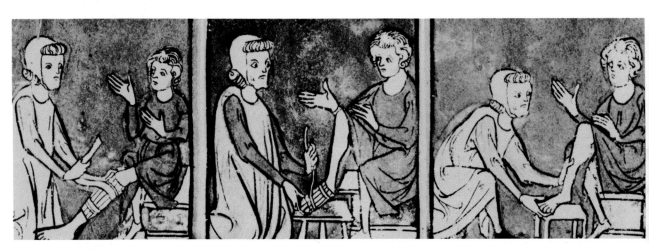

Fig 2.2　Splinting of leg and foot from medieval manuscript. (By courtesy of the Wellcome Trustees.)

the ages. Some are curious, some theoretically beneficial and some plain revolting. The excreta of animals was a lasting favourite and one wonders how much tetanus and anthrax was caused in this way over the centuries. Milk was a great favourite for washing wounds, as was human urine, in urgent situations such as the battlefield, right up to this century; both had the merit of being about the only sterile fluids readily available.

Honey was another substance in the same class, its use being consistently recommended over several thousands of years; again it was relatively free from pathogens and was obviously a bland and plastic emollient. Dust and earth, tree-bark and ashes, rags and paper, oils and tar, powdered leaves – especially juniper and solanum, butter and fats . . . the list is almost endless, being more related to availability and changing fashions than to any 'double-blind clinical trials' to test their effectiveness.

DOCUMENTATION

The first written records of medical and surgical techniques come from Ancient Egypt, where two famous medical papyri, as well as some tomb and temple hieroglyphics, give us much detail about wound treatment several thousand years before Christ.

All types of injuries are described, for instance, a broken nose was treated by inserting two greased plugs of linen up the nostrils and splinting the exterior by rolls of stiff linen. A comminuted fracture of the skull was given a local application of crushed ostrich egg in grease, the poultice being bandaged in position for three days, after which, rather optimistically, the skull would have healed, 'the colour being similar to that of the ostrich egg'. This is obviously a case of sympathetic magic, the smooth dome of the large egg being chosen for its similarity to a skull.

Lacerations were sewn together and a dressing of fresh meat bound over them – a forerunner of the modern beef-steak cure for a bruised eye. If a wound tore open after primary stitch-

ing, the Egyptian doctors directed that a second attempt should be made by sealing two strips of linen over the gash, which should then be treated daily with the popular mixture of honey and grease spread on the lint – the first mention of a dressing fabric that has been in use for over 4000 years.

The surgical records from along the Nile describe probing wounds, removing foreign bodies and bone fragments, as well as adhesive plasters for bringing wound edges together — a very distant forerunner of our Elastoplast and Bandaids!

Only slightly later, surgeons in Sumeria and Babylon were equally active. Some of our knowledge of them comes from a stone pillar carved on the orders of King Hammurabi in about 1900 BC. This describes penalties for surgical negligence; if a doctor successfully opened an ophthalmic abscess, he was paid a fixed rate, but if the patient died, the surgeon had his hands cut off — so probably he chose his patients with considerable care!

Hindu surgery was very advanced in the centuries leading up to the time of Christ and is recorded in the writings of famous surgeons like Susruta. Again, bandages and poultices were a favourite treatment for wounds. Plastic surgery, especially rhinoplasty, was performed, the latter being very popular as one common punishment for crime was cutting off the nose.

Moving back to Europe, the great doctors of ancient times were, of course, the Greeks — even Roman medicine later owed most of its surgical expertise to the Greeks who formed the majority of Rome's civil and military doctors. Hippocrates, the father of medicine, went in for simple regimes in wound treatment, typically several thousand years ahead of his time. Using bland dressings in contrast to the weird and wonderful fads of his predecessors, he felt that it was best to let nature do the healing, unhindered by meddlesome ointments.

Hippocrates taught that the wound edges should be kept dry and brought together as closely as possible to allow 'healing by first intention'. This phrase meant healing without sepsis, so different to the decline of later years,

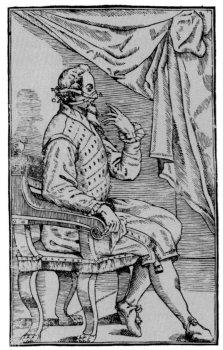

Fig 2.3 Rhinoplasty, showing early bandaging techniques, 1597. (By courtesy of the Wellcome Trustees.)

when right up to the antiseptic advances of the 19th century, it was thought that suppuration was essential to healing. The very description 'laudable pus' conjures up the approval of surgeons for stinking, septic wounds that befouled hospital wards for hundreds of years.

INSTRUMENTS, DRESSINGS AND TECHNIQUES

Largely due to their great legionary army, the Romans had highly advanced surgery — especially considering that there was no anaesthesia apart from alcohol and opium. Surgery was offered for cataracts, breast cancer, hernias, urinary stones, tonsils and many other conditions. The range of surgical instruments, such as those found in military hospitals and at Pompeii, would not have been out of place in a modern operating theatre. The wounds of both elective surgery and battle casualties were treated energetically, being irrigated with wine,

sea-water and oil and poulticed with bread, wheat and many other substances. Salts of copper and other metals were used as astringents and figs were bound over ulcerating lesions. This procedure has a scientific basis, as the enzyme papain in figs can dissolve the slough in the wound.

In the long medieval period, medicine and surgery declined, the fall of the Roman Empire and the tyranny of the Church stifling scientific advances for a thousand years. The remnants of Greek learning were carried through the Dark Ages by the Arabian physicians, but many of the more rational procedures were lost in favour of semi-magical rituals.

The doctrine of 'laudable pus', mentioned earlier, was introduced in late Roman times by the great Galen and his writings were misinterpreted and slavishly followed for centuries. Wounds were tortured to make them septic, even if they had been clean at the start. Cauterising and searing with hot irons, packing the wounds to keep them open and applying all sorts of ridiculous salves and ointments defeated nature's attempts to effect simple healing.

Several famous doctors, such as Henri de Mondeville in the 13th century and Paracelsus in the 16th, tried to return to Hippocrates' methods, but their reactionary colleagues, overawed by the long-dead Galen, and his champion, the Church, persisted in meddlesome tampering with wounds until the scientific revolution of Pasteur and Lister in the 19th century.

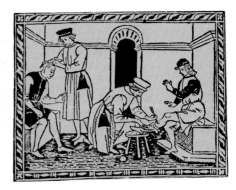

Fig 2.4 Surgical scene; woodcut c. 1490. (By courtesy of the Wellcome Trustees.)

Soldiers wounded on the battlefields of the Middle Ages suffered far more from the hands of their surgeons than from their original wounds. Especially after the introduction of gunpowder, such wounds were treated barbar- ically. They were cauterised with red-hot metal and instruments were devised to hold open the edges so that boiling oil could be injected from specially-made syringes.

The founder of military surgery in the 1500s

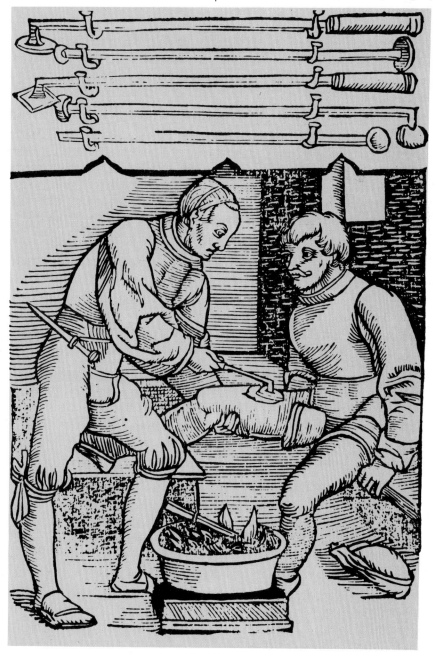

Fig 2.5 Cauterising a wound; woodcut from a manual of field surgery, 1593. (By courtesy of Ann Ronan Picture Library and E.P. Goldschmidt & Co.)

was Ambroise Paré but, unfortunately, he was a 'laudable pus' enthusiast, although it seems his writings were worse than his actual technique. In one battle, he ran out of boiling oil and was forced to use egg-yolks. He was surprised to find that his mortality rate dropped dramatically and he then gave up burning the wounds of the victims of gunshots.

The English soldiers at the Battle of Crecy in 1346 carried boxes of spiderwebs to lay across their wounds, this being a treatment for bleeding that has persisted into recent times in rural areas. Shakespeare mentions it in *Midsummer Night's Dream* and in *King Lear*; another of his many medical references describes the use of flax and egg-white for a bleeding face wound.

The material of dressings has its own specific history. Linen and flax were the most popular for a long time, but wool, tow, cotton and flannel were also employed. Strangely, many references to wool show a preference for 'dirty wool', perhaps because it was softer. Until the advent of antisepsis, dressings were used over and over again, even though they might have been drenched in pus. They were usually washed between patients, mainly to soften them again, but the concept of sterility was unknown and cross-infection was inevitable – although as sepsis was encouraged, no one noticed!

INTO THE TWENTIETH CENTURY

The greatest advance in wound treatment is almost too well known to be described. Once Louis Pasteur had made his remarkable discoveries about micro-organisms, the rationale of first antiseptic and then aseptic surgery was understood. The carbolic spray of Joseph Lister was an absolute necessity to follow the discovery and use of anaesthesia by surgeons like his near-namesake Robert Liston. Between the 1840s and 1870s, surgery was revolutionised and the longer operating times made possible by anaesthesia allowed a longer period for infection to occur in contrast with the earlier 'smash-and-grab' techniques that were necessary when the victims were conscious.

From antisepsis, with its secondary risks of tissue necrosis from phenol, it was a much quicker step to asepsis, and modern surgery and wound care revolves totally around this concept. Dressings became sterile, as well as surgeon's hands and their procedures. New materials were developed for special purposes, for example, the First World War saw 'tulle gras' introduced by the French surgeon Lumière. For a time in the same war and even in the Second World War, sphagnum-moss dressings were in vogue, but were largely replaced by cotton.

The modern history of dressings and wound treatment follows the almost explosive expansion of scientific knowledge, the greatest advance of this century being the advent of antibiotics, used both systemically or by application to the wound itself by insufflation or incorporation into the dressing material. Simplicity in wound treatment has come full circle from Hippocrates, with both transparent and porous films being used, or even complete exposure under sterile conditions.

We have come a long way since it took Ambroise Paré two years of bribery to get the secrets of a new salve for gunshot wounds from a surgeon in Turin. This special balm was made by boiling newly-born puppies in oil of lilies and adding earth-worms in turpentine. With surgeons like that, what patient needed enemies?

Chapter 3

Fundamentals of Wound Healing

Stephen Westaby

The process of wound repair is a normal reaction to injury and the keystone on which modern surgery is founded. The formation of scar tissue occurs through a series of cellular and biochemical processes. This orderly sequence (Fig 3.1) has only recently been fully understood though historically most fundamental advances in wound care have coincided with new insights into the reparative mechanism.

In the pioneering days of de Chauliac, Paré and Lister wound infections occured with such regularity as to be considered a routine phase of wound healing. The appearance of pus was regarded as a sign that eventual repair might be expected and when Semmelweiss, Lister and others worked to show that sepsis had an adverse effect on healing they were ostracised for their unorthodox thinking. Fortunately, refinements in surgical technique primarily with antiseptic skin preparation, and secondarily with the advent of antibiotics, now make sepsis the exception rather than the rule.

To a lesser extent surgeons have still not grappled fully with the inevitability of scarring. Just as early surgeons expected sepsis, surgeons today accept scarring. Some scarring is a biological necessity, though certain operative sequelae such as keloid, hypertropic scars, puncture marks and cross-hatching from skin sutures should be avoidable. Progress in this field requires an understanding of the normal process of wound repair and the best setting for this is a healthy patient with a normal vascular system. In the clinical situation this is not always the case and consideration must also be given to the influence of disease and poor general condition on wound healing.

HEALING – THE NORMAL MECHANISM

It is convenient to describe the local process of wound healing in four stages although, in reality, this is a continuous process with one stage merging into the next.

Stage I: The phase of traumatic inflammation (0–3 days)

This stage demonstrates all the features of acute inflammation due to infection and hence the confusion historically. Infection plays no part however. Redness, swelling and local heat occur in a recent wound as part of normal healing. This phase begins within a few minutes of wounding and lasts for about 3 days. When tissue is disrupted, blood vessels are injured and bleed into the space created. Platelets and the coagulation system cause blood to clot the wound. Injured blood vessels thrombose and bleeding stops. Damaged tissue and mast cells secrete histamine and other enzymes causing vasodilation of surrounding capillaries and exudation of serum and white cells into the damaged area. This increased blood supply with oedema and engorgement of

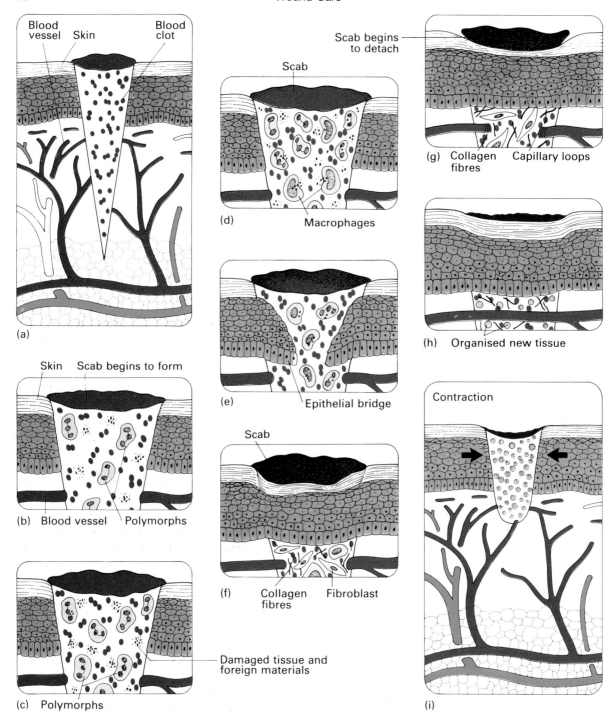

Fig 3.1 Hour-by-hour view of the wound healing process (primary intention). (a) Immediately following surgery; (b) 2 hours postsurgery; (c) 6 hours postsurgery; (d) 12 hours postsurgery; (e) 24 hours postsurgery; (f) 48 hours postsurgery; (g) 6 days postsurgery; (h) 2 weeks postsurgery; (i) At 3 to 4 days contraction reduces the area of a wound with tissue loss.

surrounding vessels accounts for the inflammatory appearance, warmth and throbbing sensation experienced by the patient. This is a purely beneficial reaction and there is no advantage in attempting to cool the area or reduce swelling unless this occurs in a closed compartment where important structures may be compressed (as in the neck or closed fascial compartments).

At this stage, two important cell types arrive in the wound. Polymorphoneucleocytes and macrophages serve to combine in defence against bacteria and begin the process of repair by clearing debris, damaged tissue, and blood clot. If too little inflammation occurs, the reparative process is slow as after steroid administration or debilitating disease. If too much, the repair process is prolonged since excessive numbers of cells compete for available nutrition. A prolonged inflammatory phase also delays formation of new tissue and thus results in retarded development of tensile strength as shown in Fig 3.2. A heightened inflammatory reaction can sometimes be avoided by removing local factors which predispose to inflammation. These include traumatised or devitalised tissue, foreign bodies or excess suture material. Poor technique when handling the wound will

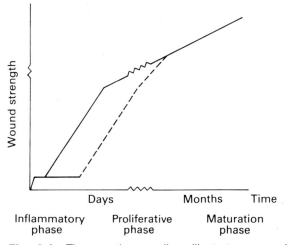

Fig 3.2 The continuous line illustrates normal strength development in a wound; the broken line shows the principal alteration in case of a prolonged inflammatory phase.

also tend to increase the inflammatory response and prolong its duration.

Stage II: The destructive phase (2–5 days)

Here the polymorphs and macrophages clear the wound of devitalised and unwanted material. Macrophages are large mobile cells with the ability to engulf and digest bacteria and dead tissue. They are found in the best and worst vascularised tissues and in tissue spaces such as the peritoneal cavity. The process of repair occurs unabated even with major reductions in the number of polymorphs in a clean wound, but if the macrophage is eliminated, healing stops. This is probably because they act as 'director' cells attracting further macrophage migration and stimulating the formation and multiplication of fibroblasts – the cell which synthesises collagen. Collagen is the body's principal structural protein and can be found in fresh wounds as soon as the 2nd day.

A simple experiment illustrates the role of the macrophage in the orchestration of wound repair. Macrophages can be extracted from a healing wound and placed into the cornea of the eye which normally has no blood vessels. Corneal cells are stimulated to form fibroblasts which, in turn, synthesise collagen fibres. The cornea then becomes vascularised by ingrowth of new blood vessels from the surrounding tissues in a process which resembles wound healing. In Stage II, therefore, macrophages play an important role by recruiting fibroblasts as well as clearing unwanted debris. New blood vessels grow into the wound from the edges and fibroblasts follow them to assume their role, analogous to construction workers after the demolition squad clears the site.

There is great cellular activity and enzymatic breakdown of unwanted fibrin and dead cells brought about by macrophage and polymorph lysosomal contents discharged into the area. The smaller protein molecules produced by enzymatic degradation convey an increased osmolality to the area and attract more water by osmosis. The obligatory swelling of the part therefore increases and may in itself prove dangerous in a restricted compartment, for instance, following fracture of the tibia where the muscles, nerves and blood vessels are contained within a restrictive fascial compartment (or plaster of Paris). Compression of these structures results in an ischaemic numb leg requiring fasciotomy. It is important to understand the mechanism of such problems and consequently anticipate them.

With the appearance of new blood vessels and multiplication of fibrolasts, Stage III begins.

Stage III: The proliferative (or fibroplasia) phase (3–24 days)

A semblance of order appears in the wound on the 3rd day in a healthy patient. Fibroblasts line up behind the macrophages and begin to produce the strands of collagen which is the main constituent of skin, tendons, ligaments, bones, cartilage, fascia and scar tissue. The peak rate of synthesis of new collagen in a primarily healing wound occurs on about the 5th to the 7th day (Fig 3.3). Early collagen is highly disorganised and its synthesis depends to a critical degree on the vascularity and the extent to which the circulatory system perfuses the wound. Fibroblasts need stimulation to

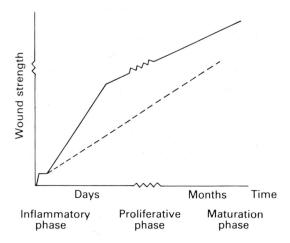

Fig 3.3 The continuous line illustrates normal wound strength development; the broken line shows the principal alteration in impaired fibroplasia.

produce collagen and this happens best in a slightly acid environment.

The most prominent stimulators are vitamin C and lactate ions which accumulate in areas of low oxygen concentration as in the centre of the wound. The fibroblast itself is a hardy cell which can survive the most hostile environments, but without vitamin C collagen synthesis is inhibited whereas breakdown continues. Two of the principal effects of scurvy are breakdown of unsupported blood vessels with bleeding (purpura) and failure of new wounds to heal (Fig 3.4). Since the body cannot store vitamin C the importance of adequate nutrition in this stage of wound healing is apparent.

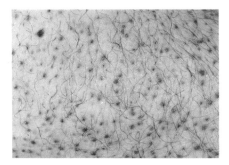

Fig 3.4 Purpura caused by vitimin C deficiency.

This considerable cellular and chemical activity during the proliferative phase results in the formation of 'granulation tissue'. This used to be known as 'proud flesh' and consists of new and fragile capillary loops supported in a scaffolding of collagen fibres. The amount of granulation tissues produced depends to an extent on the amount of inflammation (Stage I).

Too much inflammation may lead to excessive granulation and to an increased production of scar tissue (hypertrophic scar). Retained dead tissue, foreign bodies, wound infection or excessive suture material all increase inflammation and intensify the degree of fibroblastic proliferation so that the end result is an excessive amount of scar tissue.

As the proliferative phase proceeds there is a rapid increase in the tensile strength of the wound (it takes more force to destract the wound edges) as a scaffolding of collagen is laid down progressively. It is important that movement is minimised so as to protect the delicately oriented new fibres. In as much as the fibroblastic process is non specific, the increase in strength is similar in all wounds. This means that the strength of the wound in relation to the strength of the surrounding intact tissue varies considerably. For example, an intestinal anastomosis can be stronger than the intact intestine after only 7 days, while at this time an incision in fascia or skin has reached only a small part of the strength of the intact tissue. Most of the factors that impair healing during this period are systemic and include age, oxygen tension, anaemia, hypoproteinaemia and zinc deficiency. Nevertheless, it is important to recognise these factors since wounds with a decreased healing rate require prolonged suture support.

Although the signs of inflammation successively subside during this phase, the wound remains red, raised and often itchy.

Stage IV: The maturation phase (24 days – 1 year)

During this stage there is a progressive decrease in vascularity of the scar, shrinkage of the fibroblasts, enlargement and reorientation of the collagen fibres and augmentation of tensile strength. This is when the dusky red appearance of vascular granulation tissue changes to the pale white avascular scar tissue with which we are familiar.

While the strength of the wound increases rapidly from the 6th to the 21st day, only 50% of the normal tensile stength of a skin wound is regained within the first 6 weeks, and in all healing tissues the amount of collagen in the scar increases for several months. It then gradually reduces causing the well-known flattening and softening of the incision as the scar matures.

Tension in the wound produces profound changes in orientation of the collagen fibres so that they lie at right angles to the wound margins. Increased tension also causes more col-

lagen to be laid down and if the healing wound is examined under the microscope at this stage, the overall effect appears to be one of lacing the wound edges together with a three-dimensional weave.

In addition to the four cellular and chemical phases described above, there are two other mechanisms to be considered. These are the processes of contraction and epithelisation which are of the greatest importance when there has been tissue loss or destruction (as in avulsion injury or burns).

Contraction

Contraction is the process by which large wounds become small without the need for secondary closure or skin graft. This allows us to leave a contaminated wound wide open, yet healing occurs almost as rapidly as if the wound were sutured.

In 1793 John Hunter wrote: 'In the amputation of the thick thigh (which is naturally seven, eight or more inches in diameter) . . . the cicatrix shall be no broader than a crown piece (1.5 inches).' Thus 90% of the amputation wound was closed by centripetal movement of the wound edges. Amputation wounds are seldom left open these days so let us consider a more familiar situation – a rectangular piece of full thickness skin is excised to remove a malignant melanoma. The skin edges are freely moveable and their natural elasticity causes them to contract so that the wound will first become larger. After 3 or 4 days the wound area begins to decrease as the original edges move towards the centre. Eventually after about 3 weeks they meet, leaving a linear scar in the shape of two Ys, tail to tail. Wounds that heal by contracture usually heal with a good functional and cosmetic result — (Fig 3.5).

There are, however, areas of the body where contraction gives a poor result. Wounds of the lower leg that are fixed closely to the tibia will not close by contraction. Wounds on the face will contract, but because the skin is fixed to so many structures nearby, there is a purse-string effect and distortion of the features will result.

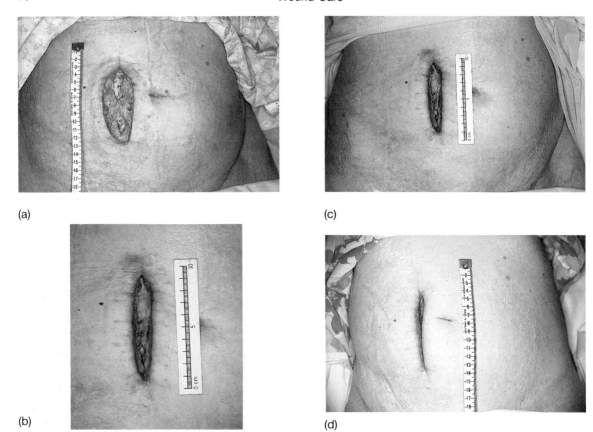

(a)

(b)

(c)

(d)

Fig 3.5 (a)–(d)   Healing by secondary intention of a dehisced laporotomy wound.

On the other hand, on the back of the neck, abdomen and breasts even the largest wounds close with small scars. The mechanism of wound contracture is not clearly understood. However, certain facts are known and these are:

* Collagen is not essential.
* The motive force for contraction comes from a cell and any event which interferes with the viability of cells at the wound edge will inhibit contraction.
* The cells that supply the motive force appear to be a special type of contractile cell having attributes of both the fibroblast and smooth muscle cell. These cells have been called myofibroblasts. Contraction begins on about the 4th day and proceeds side by side with epithelisation and the cellular and biochemical processes of wound healing.

Epithelisation

Skin has a covering of squamous epithelial cells which are constantly being shed and replaced from below. When a defect is made in the squamous covering, the cells at the wound edge multiply, flatten and migrate towards the area of cell deficit. This migration begins within hours of wounding during the stage of traumatic inflammation. Epithelial cells will only migrate over live tissue and, therefore, the cells move into the layer below the debris, blood clot or eschar (scab).

The same process occurs in the micro wound created by skin sutures and results in the puncture site scars and occasionally 'inclusion cysts' which appear at the side of the principal wound. This is one reason why skin sutures should be avoided where possible. Extensive superficial injuries such as second degree burns epithelise not only from the wound edge, but from hair follicles and other deep dermal appendages that supply live squamous cells.

The intensive cellular activity at the edge of an open wound produces a thickened, active looking hyperplastic zone that disappears when epithelisation is complete. This may occur as quickly as 24 hours in the incised wound. The final epithelial scar is thick, flat and often ridged because epithelisation is usually accompanied by contraction.

In wounds with tissue loss allowed to heal by secondary intention, the protective influence of a scab or surgical dressing prevents physical trauma, drying, haemorrhage and contact with foreign material while the delicate epithelial cells cut their path over viable tissue beneath.

Successful epithelisation occurs only if the cumulative effects of physical manipulation, drying, bacterial enzymes, wound area and limitation of blood supply do not exceed the capacity for available cells to divide and move across the surface. A moist environment is preferable in this respect and although epithelisation will occur under dry dressings, it proceeds at a considerably slower rate.

The process of epithelisation is of great importance in the study of wound healing, since the stimulus for cell division to begin after wounding and subsequently the inhibition of cell division has direct application to the study of cell behaviour in tumours. Indeed, the recognised propensity to develop cancer in certain types of wound scars (particularly radiant energy wounds such as sunburn) and in all wounds which are prevented from healing, emphasises the close similarity between cancer and the healing process. A histological section from a 5-day old healing wound can be easily interpreted as fibrosarcoma if the clinical details are not supplied.

The major difference between a healing wound and a malignant tumour is control. Cell proliferation is temporary because some regulating influence brings order out of disorder, a resting state to rapidly dividing cells, and a remodelling of recently synthesised fibrous tissue to produce a purposeful structural pattern. In many respects the controlling influence remains a mystery.

SYSTEMIC INFLUENCE

One of the oldest observations in surgery is that tissues with a poor blood supply heal slowly and are easily infected. It matters little how well nourished the patient is if essential factors cannot reach the wound because of impaired vascularity.

A healthy circulation is, therefore, of paramount importance and we might expect patients with diseased vessels, such as diabetics with atherosclerosis, to heal poorly. These problems must be taken into account when planning surgery on arteriopathic patients such as the young smoker with Buerger's disease who is well nourished, but with gangrenous extremities which show no sign of healing even after minor trauma.

It is not only large blood vessels which have importance in this context. A fundamental principle in nursing or surgery is that damaged tissues must be respected and handled gently since the more damage done to a wound the more bruising and oedema impairs the microcirculation whose integrity is essential in the early stages of the healing process.

Recently it has been observed that patients shocked after trauma, or blood loss unreplaced after surgery may manifest a considerable slowing of the healing process. Experimentally it can be shown that haemorrhage of a quite minor nature results in the withdrawal of circulation from the growing edge of healing tissue. This occurs well before a drop in blood pressure and certainly before clinically evident shock is established. Reperfusion at an early stage immediately leads to restoration of circulation to the wound. If hypovolaemia is allowed to continue to the point of shock, however, restoration of blood volume is not followed by reopening of the capillary circulation to the wound edge. This seriously impairs the healing process (Fig 3.6).

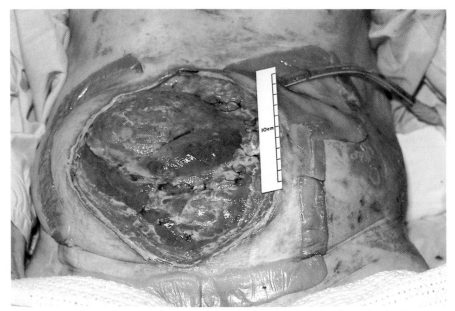

Fig 3.6 Wound dehiscence following emergency laporotomy in a shocked patient.

With the knowledge that impaired vascularity is responsible for slow healing, certain physical methods have been tried in an attempt to increase healing in refractory wounds. Infra-red rays have been shown to increase blood flow at the wound edges and promote healing.

Carbon ruby lasers and electromagnetic fields have been used to treat chronic ulcers and slowly healing bone defects and ultrasound waves have been shown to increase the healing rate and strength of suture wounds by up to 60%. The author also had some success in bypassing poor vascularity by direct irrigation of open wounds with nutrient solutions and oxygen.

Given that an adequate blood supply is essential for normal healing, another early observation was that starved patients heal poorly and the better the general condition of the patient the better the state of the wound. While it is unusual to encounter a patient suffering from malnutrition in our environment, it is important to remember that there are many other reasons for starvation in an otherwise well-fed patient. Temporary starvation accompanies most injury, especially that of a progressive or long-term nature, and other disease processes such as malignancy, malabsorbtion syndromes, colitis or intestinal fistulae have impaired nutrient intake or excessive losses.

Which nutrients are of direct importance in wound healing? The principal structural element, collagen, is a protein assembled from amino acids acquired by the fibroblast from the products of ingested protein in food. A continued supply of protein is, therefore, essential throughout the duration of wound repair. However, with prolonged fasting in the face of injury, plasma proteins are utilised as an energy substitute in the place of depleted carbohydrate, and even muscle protein is broken down. Consequently, little is available for wound repair. Hyperalimentation or intravenous feeding with carbohydrate, fat and amino acids is then of great benefit to the injured or postoperative patient. Vitamin C is essential for collagen synthesis and has long been known to play an important role in wound repair. In addition, it has been shown that injury is accompanied by a decrease in plasma vitamin C levels. Consequently, intravenous administration of large doses has been recommended after operation. Other vitamins have also been

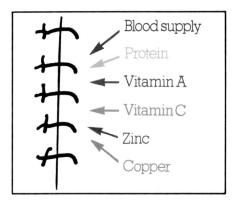

Fig 3.7 Substances which encourage wound healing.

found to be of direct importance (Fig 3.7). Certain types of trauma, such as burns, are accompanied by a decrease in blood and liver concentrations of vitamin A and this, in turn, is associated with stress induced peptic ulcers. Restoration of vitamin A levels markedly reduces the risk of ulceration. Collagen synthesis and wound healing are suppressed by steroid hormones, but it is now evident that this can be returned to normal by vitamin A administration.

Although the role of trace elements in wound repair requires clearer definition, there is increasing evidence that zinc and copper are essential for normal healing. Zinc is necessary for both epithelisation and collagen synthesis, but while zinc depletion slows wound healing, this process cannot be speeded up by giving zinc to individuals with normal levels. Copper is an essential component of an enzyme that links collagen fibres. Drugs which bind copper (penicillamine) are chemically useful for treatment of diseases characterised by overabundant collagen disposition, such as cirrhosis, keloid formation, scleroderma or oesophageal stricture.

It is important to maintain a balanced nutritional supply to the wounded patient whether this be by the oral or intravenous route. Only in this way will the basic building materials for normal wound healing be kept in adequate supply and without these materials active healing stops. When one considers the numerous

disease processes in which wound healing is characteristically impaired (Table 1), this is virtually always as a result of poor vascularity or inadequate availability of essential nutrient factors.

In addition, special care must be taken in the treatment of even minor cuts and abrasions in a few rare congenital conditions such as the Ehlers-Danlos syndrome where collagen synthesis and scar tissue formation are impaired. Fortunately, these are only rarely encountered in clinical practice. It is well known that infection delays healing. When organisms are introduced into a wound, they modify the local environment to a considerable extent. Aerobic bacteria have a high oxygen consumption which detracts from that available for the rapidly proliferating cells. Collagen synthesis may therefore be slowed. Diseases such as diabetes or rheumatoid arthritis which predispose to infection are commonly associated with poor healing.

Three types of medication are commonly considered to adversely influence the rate of healing in patients receiving them. Firstly anti-

Table 1
CONDITIONS ASSOCIATED WITH POOR WOUND HEALING

Vascular disorders	*Decreased resistance to infection*
Arteriosclerosis	Diabetes
Buerger's disease	Immune disorders
Raynaud's and other	Chronic infection
vascular diseases	Drug therapy; steroids;
Diabetes	cytotixics;
	antimicrobials
Poor nutritional state	*Miscellaneous*
Malignancy	Elderly
Protein loosing	Obesity
eneropathy	Radiation therapy
Inflammatory bowel	Cushing's disease
disease	Addison's disease
Hepatic failure	Rheumatoid arthritis
Renal failure	
Autoimmune disorders	

Many conditions affect repair through more than one mechanism

inflammatory drugs theoretically might suppress the important phase of acute inflammation. Drugs such as aspirin, phenylbutazone or salazopryrine, in fact, have a negligible influence in ordinary therapeutic doses and may be given for relief of pain or to lower temperature without fear of adverse effects.

The effects of steroids have been debated for many years; classically steroids were thought to delay healing, and, if administered in large doses continuously, this may well be the case. When present before injury they supress multiplication of fibroblasts and this influence is enhanced by starvation or protein deficiency. By damping the immunological reaction to infection, steroids also predispose to wound infection. However, the outpouring of one's own steroid hormones by the stress of trauma has little influence on healing and neither do single doses given after injury. Anabolic steroids stimulate protein synthesis and in this way may increase the rate of repair.

Cytotoxic drugs (nitrogen mustard, vincristine, bleomycin and so on) used in the treatment of malignant disease interfere with cell proliferation and have the capacity to seriously impair healing and reduce tensile strength. This may be important after operation for malignant tumours when it is desirable to kill cancer cells spread by manipulation.

The author once used cytotoxic drugs for preoperative treatment of lung cancer patients. When the sutures were removed from their incisions after lung resection, the wounds dehisced with no sign of healing. In this circumstance it is difficult to weigh the dangers of wound dehiscence against the potential benefits of cancer chemotherapy. As in many forms of medical treatment some form of compromise is desirable.

THE SCAR AND ABNORMALITIES OF WOUND HEALING

All accidental wounds and surgical incisions leave a permanent reminder of the event in the form of a scar, the inevitable end point of the wound healing process. All scars pass through the following of stages.

Stage I:
0–4 weeks   The scar is soft, fine and weak.
Stage II:
4–12 weeks   The scar contracts, becoming red, hard, thick and strong.
Stage III
12–40 weeks The scar gradually becomes soft, supple, white and loose.

The outcome of scarring is to some extent age and race dependent. In infancy (first 12 months) scars resolve quickly with minimal residual effect. After 12 months scarring becomes more marked and the worst period for producing unsightly contracted scars is in late childhood. Old people with thin wrinkled skin may heal poorly, but their scars settle quickly without contraction and disfigurement. The more highly pigmented the skin the worse the scars will be, hence the influence of race. Extreme hypertrophy of scar is common in deeply pigmented Negroes. Scars are better when they occur in the natural lines of skin tension that is lying in or parallel with natural skin folds. Scars which directly cross skin folds, particularly flexion creases of joints become exaggerated and their contraction may restrict joint movement, especially after burns. Scars on the trunk tend to be worse than those on limbs. The worst positions are over the sternum, shoulder and upper back.

The area and extent of scarring are principally determined within the first 12 weeks. Hypertrophic scars are common in young people particularly after severe burns. Here the active phase of scar formation is increased and the area becomes thick, red and itchy. Even with severe hypertrophy, the size of the scar does not increase after 12 weeks but the irritation may persist for 3–6 months. Hypertrophic scars are always confined within the original area of the wound and are more common in women than men. The cause is unknown, but the strain across the wound is one important factor.

Keloid scarring is different from hypertrophic scarring in that the process sometimes continues for as long as 5–10 years and may spread into surrounding normal tissue not affected by the original injury or operation. Natural stabilisation of the collagen fibres appears to be inhibited. True keloid formation is extremely rare in white skinned races and probably occurs only on the sternum. Malignant changes with development of fibrosarcoma is extremely rare, but may occur in any scar, often many years after original formation. Foreign bodies within the wound may predispose to this. These adversely affect the course of wound healing by creating a chronic inflammatory reaction. Gravel is often driven into the subcutaneous tissues of the face, hands or knees during road accidents and results in unsightly pigmentation. In all but minor cases meticulous removal with a stiff brush under anaesthetic is advisable. Pieces of clothing are commonly driven deep into penetrating wounds particularly after shotgun injuries. All clothing is contaminated with bacteria and bacterial spores and should be removed. Glass usually contains enough lead to be radiopaque and every laceration or puncture wound caused by glass should be examined radiologically and retained fragments removed.

Implantation dermoid cysts may arise from squamous epithelium which has been driven beneath the skin by penetration. Suture of skin incisions drives small bits of epidermis into the subcutaneous layers and increases the incidence of wound infection as compared with sutureless skin closure. Stitch abscesses occur in connection with percutaneous sutures, most often when silk and braided synthetic materials are used.

Subcutaneous knots of non-absorbable suture material may be painful, irritating and eventually ulcerate, so absorbable materials are best in this situation. A suture granuloma is a painful swelling related to a buried suture or ligature and may result from infection, mechanical or chemical irritation. Sinus formation may follow. With thought, care and appropriate treatment, there is much that can be done to minimise the risks of unsightly scarring or poor wound healing.

Chapter 4

The Surgical Incision and Haemostasis

William S. Fountain and Stephen Westaby

When planning a surgical incision, three principal factors should be taken into account. First the incision must give access to the site of the operation. Second the incision must be able to heal afterwards and third it must leave as good a cosmetic effect as can be obtained within the limits of the other factors concerned.

Before considering incisions in terms of their anatomical site and the part played by these factors in choosing individual incisions, it is perhaps appropriate to discuss each factor in general.

Access

In surgery, access is all. The principal purpose of any incision must be to obtain access to the operative site, and that is as true for an operation to remove a subcutaneous cyst from the leg as it is for a heart transplant. The ease with which access can be obtained depends on the structure or organ to be operated on and its anatomical site, but it should always be the first and most important consideration to be taken into account.

Ideally, the best access is obtained by making the incision directly over the site. A compromise is sometimes made, in specific areas, for the sake of cosmesis, but in operations on the chest or abdomen, such compromises are rarely justifiable.

Apart from being directly over the site, the ideal incision must also be of adequate length

and it should be extendable at both ends. However comprehensive preoperative investigations may have been, the full extent of any operative procedure can only be decided at operation itself.

Wound healing

Clearly the way in which a wound heals depends mainly on the manner and circumstances of its closure, but the incision plays a vital part in wound healing as well. Skin and all deeper tissues will heal best if cut cleanly with a knife at right angles to the tissue plane.

Cutting diathermy with a sharp point can be used to cut through large muscle masses with considerable saving in time and blood loss because it coagulates blood vessels as it cuts, but anything which causes trauma to wound edges — be it blunt scissors or blades, over-zealous stripping of tissue planes by hand or excessive use of coagulation diathermy — may lead to poor healing and wound infection.

Cosmetic effect

The direction of natural skin creases is important partly because incisions made parallel to, or in, skin creases heal better, and partly because they leave a finer and, therefore, more cosmetic scar. In 1861, Professor Karl Langer of Vienna described natural lines of skin cleavage now known as Langer's lines (Fig 4.1). His discovery was based on the fact that sub-

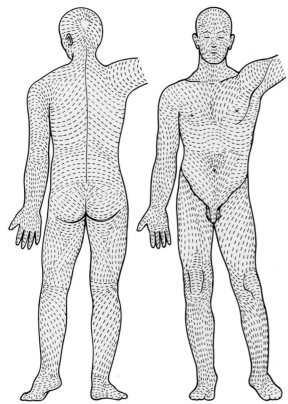

Fig 4.1 Langer's lines.

cutaneous collagen fibres are disposed in parallel bundles in the human body and thus skin which is breached will split preferentially along the direction of these bundles rather in the manner that cloth, when torn, will split along the weave.

Lines of skin tension generally follow the direction of Langer's lines as do, therefore, natural skin creases. Incisions made along these creases will tend to fall together and incisions made across them will tend to gape apart, hence their importance to wound healing and scar appearance.

ABDOMINAL INCISIONS

Access

The incision will obviously depend on the structure or organ to be operated on (Fig 4.2). Vertical incisions are historically more popu-

lar than oblique or transverse incisions because they are extendable. The abdomen is notoriously 'full of surprises' and although modern methods of investigation make abdominal operations more predictable than formerly, if any doubt exists in the surgeon's mind as to the extent of exposure required, a vertical incision allows potential access to any intra- or retroperitoneal structure.

Emergency laparotomies are therefore nearly always performed through some kind of vertical incision. For elective procedures, oblique or transverse incisions may be used.

A right subcostal, or Kocher's incision is commonly used for operations on the gallbladder and a Rutherford Morrison, right or left inferior oblique, for resections of the right or left colon. Transverse incisions are becoming more popular.

Good access to the prostate gland in a man or the uterus in a woman can be obtained with a suprapubic skin crease or Pfannenstiel incision. The pancreas and portal venous system

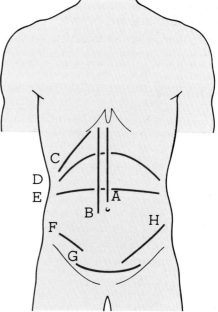

Fig 4.2 Abdominal incisions. A = midline epigastric; B = right paramedian; C = right subcostal (Kocher's); D = bilateral subcostal; E = transverse epigastric; F = gridiron (McBurney's); G = transverse suprapubic (Pfannenstiel); H = left inferior oblique (Rutherford Morrison).

as well as the stomach and gastro-oesophageal junction can be easily reached through a transverse epigastric or bilateral subcostal incision.

Wound healing

Much has been written and more has been said about the relative merits of different abdominal incisions with respect to their healing properties. Vertical incisions may be in the midline or to the right or left of it (paramedian incisions). Midline incisions provide quick access since all the muscle sheaths of the abdominal wall are condensed in the midline to form the thick fibrous and relatively avascular linea alba (Fig 4.3).

Paramedian incisions divide the anterior and posterior rectus sheaths separately. The muscle itself is traditionally peeled off the medial part of the sheath and retracted laterally, a time-consuming business in an emergency, but the muscle itself may be split or incised in the direction of its fibres in the so-called rectus splitting incision.

Protagonists of the traditional paramedian incision claim that repairing the anterior and posterior muscle sheaths separately produces a stronger wound than can be achieved with the one layer closure of a midline incision and that the rectus splitting incision devitalises the muscle on the medial side of the wound.

In fact, not one of these incisions has shown itself to be innately superior to another and all three are commonly performed so it is unlikely that these considerations are of vital importance.

Cosmetic effect

It will be apparent immediately that the commonly performed vertical abdominal incisions run across lines of skin tension and, therefore, leave thick, and often unsightly, scars. This is because, historically, access has overriden other considerations in abdominal surgery. Extending transverse or skin crease incisions is often difficult or unhelpful, or both, but so long as the required exposure can be obtained, such incisions are usually superior in terms of wound healing and cosmetic effect.

A special word ought to be said about the most commonly performed abdominal incision because it seems to transgress so many of the views so far espoused. The gridiron incision is difficult to extend and splits muscle, causing local trauma. It offers access only to a normally placed appendix and, if performed more laterally in the skin crease, even that can be difficult. It is, nevertheless, an entirely satisfactory incision for simple appendicectomy and, considering the high rate of wound infection associated with appendicitis, it heals well.

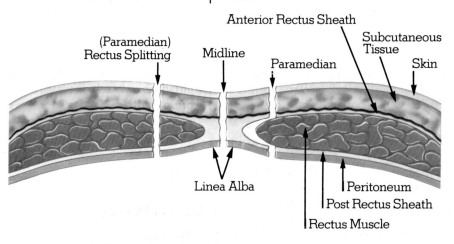

Fig 4.3 Abdominal incisions (transverse section).

THORACIC INCISIONS

Access

The number of routes of access to the pleural cavities and mediastinum is limited by the configuration of the bony chest wall (Fig 4.4). Thus operations on the lung, pleura and oesophagus, as well as some 'closed' cardiac procedures are performed by incising between two ribs and spreading them apart. The skin incision used follows roughly the direction of the interspace to be divided. Thoracotomies are more often posterolateral than anterolater-

routinely performed through such an incision and on the right, the middle third of the oesophagus is also accessible.

The descending aorta on the left is best reached through a fourth or fifth interspace thoracotomy, but for access to the lower third of the oesophagus and the gastro-oesophageal hiatus, a thoracotomy through the seventh left interspace is preferable. This incision can be extended across the costal margin, becoming a thoracoabdominal incision. All 'open' heart operations are carried out through a vertical midline sternotomy. The skin is incised in the midline over the length of the sternum, and

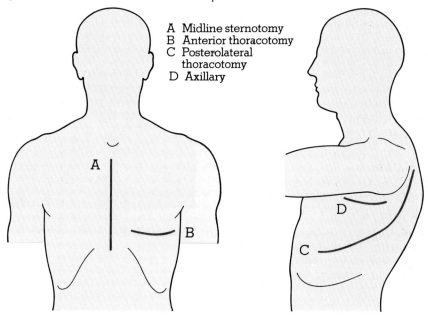

A Midline sternotomy
B Anterior thoracotomy
C Posterolateral thoracotomy
D Axillary

Fig 4.4 Thoracic incisions.

al, largely because the shape of the ribs allows them to be distracted to a greater degree posteriorly, but it is usually necessary to employ the full length of the interspace to gain sufficient access, so thoracotomies are usually long incisions.

It is best to approach the hilum of the lung through the fifth interspace – the space between the fifth and sixth rib. The incision is deepened in the line of the sixth rib dividing all the muscles of the chest wall with a knife or cutting diathermy. Lung resections are

the sternum itself is divided, usually with a vibrating saw.

This incision is a prime example of one where access overrides all other considerations as there is no other way to gain exposure of the heart sufficient to institute cardiopulmonary bypass.

Wound healing

Thoracotomy incisions generally heal well and full thickness breakdown is very uncommon.

They are necessarily long, and if damage to an intercostal nerve occurs, which it easily can, persistent pain in the scar may be a long-term problem.

The midline sternotomy, from the point of view of wound healing, is a most unsatisfactory incision. The sternum lies subcutaneously and the divided bone needs to be repaired with stout material, usually stainless steel wire. Wound sinuses are, therefore, not infrequent and infection, if it spreads to the sternum causing osteomyelitis, can be a serious complication.

Cosmetic effect

A lateral thoracotomy incision can easily be made to follow lines of skin tension without compromising access, but length is a cosmetic problem. In special circumstances, some operations, such as pleurectomy, can be performed through an axillary or submammary incision. The midline sternotomy tends to leave a thick, unsightly scar.

HEAD AND NECK INCISIONS

The skin of the face and neck has a rich blood supply and it is usually possible, by raising flaps of skin and subcutaneous tissue, to gain access to an operative site with a curved, skin crease or partly concealed incision, leaving as cosmetically satisfactory a result as possible (Fig 4.5). Operations on the skull and neurosurgical procedures on the brain can be performed through incisions behind the hairline, becoming completely concealed when the hair regrows.

Unsightly, vertical incisions on the face and neck are rarely, if ever, indicated and where a vertical component to an incision is required, as for parotidectomy, it is placed immediately in front of the ear and gradually becomes less and less noticeable. The transverse skin crease incision used for thyroidectomy eventually becomes invisible.

Because of its rich blood supply healing of

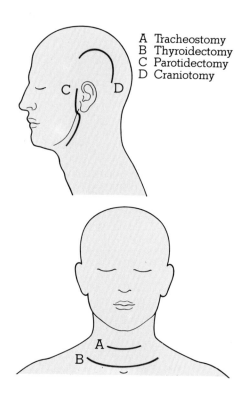

A Tracheostomy
B Thyroidectomy
C Parotidectomy
D Craniotomy

Fig 4.5 Head and neck incisions.

skin incisions of the head and neck is rapid and almost always access can be achieved with full regard to cosmetic effect. Given that all incisions leave a scar, those on the head can usually be made as inconspicuous as possible.

LIMB INCISIONS

The factors governing limb incisions are slightly different to those governing incisions elsewhere. Good access is, by and large, not a problem wherever the incision. So far as wound healing is concerned, two considerations are important. Incisions over subcutaneous bone should be avoided, if possible; they are slow to heal, often leave a thick scar and may become tethered.

An incision should never be made across the flexor surface of a joint, because as the wound heals some shortening is bound to occur, causing flexion contracture. Access to the joint can be obtained either by making the incision

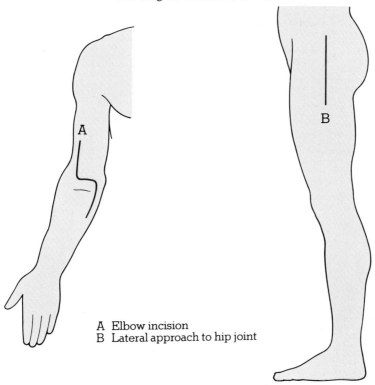

A Elbow incision
B Lateral approach to hip joint

Fig 4.6 Limb incisions.

on a lateral surface or by making an S or Z shaped incision to avoid crossing the skin crease (Fig 4.6). The importance of the cosmetic effect of limb wounds probably depends more on the individual concerned than anything else, but the guiding principles are the same as for other parts of the body.

No attempt has been made to compile an exhaustive list of surgical incisions, but some of the most common have been used to illustrate the importance of the factors governing the planning of an incision. There are, of course, other considerations to be taken into account apart from the three mentioned here when considering wounds in general, although they may not be solely dependent on the site of the incision and are therefore beyond the scope of this discussion.

It is, however, worth mentioning pain in the context of the incision, because, despite the fact that wound pain has many complex origins, it cannot be denied that the surgical incision is one of its principal causes. No incision in a normal person can be painless and the importance in recognising this is in being able to treat it adequately when it inevitably occurs. There are simple steps which can be taken when making an incision to reduce its magnitude.

Care should be taken not to divide major sensory nerves, or to burn nerves with diathermy or tie them with ligatures. Vertical incisions on the trunk may cut through three or four intercostal nerves, whereas curved or transverse incisions may divide only one or two. Closing wounds too tightly probably increases postoperative pain because tight sutures cut into tissue, an effect which is highlighted by postoperative inflammatory oedema.

It is often said that the only thing a patient remembers for ever about an operation is the scar, but it is worth remembering at the same time that this is only true if the operation is a success. A neat scar is an admirable objective in a surgeon's mind, but it must never be allowed to compromise his ability to perform a good operation.

HAEMOSTASIS

The body has its own natural haemostatic mechanisms to prevent excessive bleeding. During surgical operations or after accidental wounding the surgeon or nurse may be forced to intervene to assist these mechanisms but should not hinder them. Blood is conveyed around the circulation under pressure and when a break in continuity of the vessel wall occurs, blood will escape until there is equalisation of pressure inside and outside of the lumen or until the breach of the lumen is sealed. Equalisation of pressure may be obtained by accumulation of blood in the surrounding tissue spaces (haematoma formation) or after fall in systemic arterial pressure due to blood loss. In very large vessels fatal haemorrhage may occur unless stopped artificially by tourniquets or ligatures. However, shock and local trauma to an artery results in active constriction and there are many examples of traumatic amputation of limbs when the patient has survived despite a long interval between the event and effective help.

Most surgical and traumatic bleeding are from smaller vessels. Arterioles are contractile in response to damage and though capillaries are not, circulation through them can be obliterated by contraction at the arteriolar-capillary junction. In the normal microcirculation, there is no tendency for platelets to adhere to each other or to the endothelium. Following mechanical trauma, platelets adhere to the site and pile up by accretion, though rarely enough to block the vessel (Fig 4.7). This process effectively seals minor capillary and arteriolar defects. The platelet plug together with arteriolar vasoconstriction maintains haemostasis until the platelet plug is reinforced by the formation of fibrin. The contact of platelets with exposed collagen fibres leads to release of a number of platelet factors which stimulate further platelet aggregation (adenosine diphosphate, ADP), vasoconstriction (5-hydroxy-tryptamine) and the coagulation cascade (platelet factor 3). At an early stage the platelet plug is permeable to plasma but not to red cells. After some minutes activation of the coagulation cascade results in fibrin deposition and formation of blood clot which produces a completely haemostatic plug. The clotting process is the visible result of a chain of enzymatic reactions whereby a soluble plasma protein fibrinogen is transformed into an interlacing network of protein molecules, fibrin.

This conversion is brought about through the enzyme thrombin which splits off four small parts of the fibrinogen molecule which then polymerise into long strands of fibrin. Calcium greatly accelrates this process. Activation of thrombin from its precursor molecule prothrombin is brought about by the mechanism shown in Fig 4.8. The importance of this mechanism is demonstrated by the haemorrhagic state which accompanies severe deficiency of certain of the coagulation factors, for example factor VIII (haemophilia). In such patients dental extraction is followed by an initial phase of relative freedom from bleeding lasting 20–60 minutes when vascular contractility and platelet plug formation are functioning: when vascular contractility wears off the platelet plug is unstable since it has not been reinforced with fibrin. Bleeding ensues, is continuous and potentially life threatening without active intervention.

After formation of the haemostatic blood clot, fibroblasts grow into the plug and form a permanent connective tissue seal. This mechanism is extremely effective in normal circumstances and it is important that when bleeding from a wound has stopped, it should not be restarted by unnecessary interference. There is an old saying that 'it takes two clots to make a haemorrhage, the clot on the vessel and the clot who knocks it off'.

When major vascular damage is suspected it should be remembered that the patient is

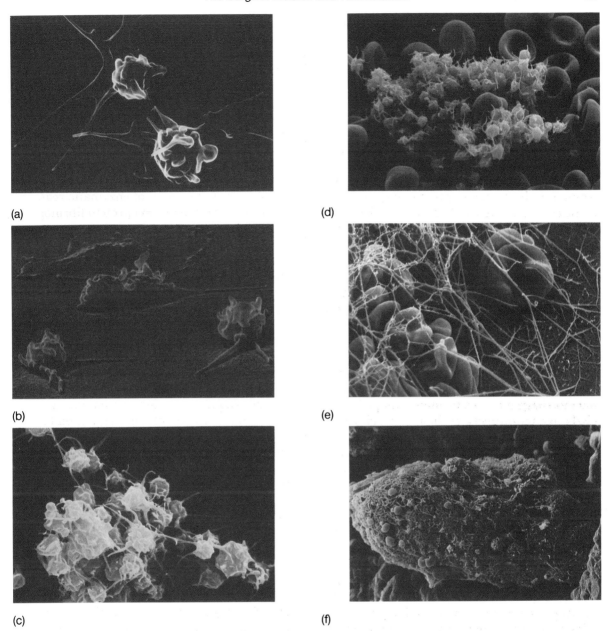

Fig 4.7 From thrombocytes to thrombosis — the platelet story. (a) When the wall of a blood vessel is subjected to insult, platelets (thrombocytes) in the vicinity respond by losing their discoid form and developing psuedopodia; (b) The psuedopodia interconnect and the platelets adhere to the injured area; (c) Platelet factors are liberated and attract more platelets to the area, producing aggregation; (d) The platelet aggregate is in intimate contact with circulating red blood cells . . . ; (e) . . . which become enmeshed, together with the platelets, in the fibrin network produced by the clotting cascade mechanism. The result is the formation of a thrombus. Venous thrombi contain more red blood cells than arterial thrombi due to the different dynamics of blood flow in veins and arteries; (f) Should thrombus formation continue unabated, a large thrombus will be produced which may project into the lumen of the vessel and obstruct the blood flow. (By courtesy of Boehringer Ingelheim)

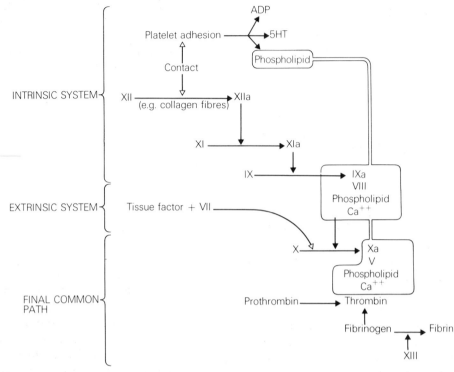

Fig 4.8 The coagulation cascade. A variety of inert precursors are present in plasma which, when stimulated, react sequentially. Two systems are present, intrinsic and extrinsic, having a final common path which leads to fibrin formation. (From *Haematology*, J.C. Cawley, ed. In *Integrated Clinical Science* series, George P. McNicol, ed. London: William Heinemann Medical Books.)

often shocked and hypotensive. Blood transfusion may restore normal blood pressure and consequently detach the haemostatic plug or overcome the occlusive vasoconstriction and resume bleeding. This commonly occurs in patients who have reached a stable state after rupture of the aorta or penetrating cardiac wounds when the surrounding haemotoma effectively prevents further bleeding until resuscitation is commenced. The precarious balance is then upset and the patient bleeds fatally.

During surgery it is impossible to rely solely on natural haemostasis which takes time. A number of different methods are, therefore, employed to expedite haemostasis as follows:

Pressure

Pressure is the simplest and most effective method for control of bleeding. Substantial compression for 5–10 minutes will frequently stop bleeding from even large vessels and may be the only satisfactory way to stem generalised capillary ooze.

Packing

On occasions it may be necessary to maintain pressure by closing the wound over packs, for instance after cardiac reoperation, liver trauma or for the diffuse pelvic venous bleeding sometimes encountered after abdomino-perineal resection of the rectum.

Clamp and ligature

A bleeding vessel is grasped cleanly with an artery forcep and a ligature applied directly to the vessel. The clamp is removed slowly so the ligature can be tightened while the vessel is still under control. Alternatively, suture ligature may be performed directly without a clamp. As an alternative to sutures, metal clips may be applied directly.

Cautery

Electrocoagulation is used both for cutting and haemostasis, but should not be used too close to the skin in order to avoid tissue gangrene and infection. This provides rapid and effective haemostasis from small bleeding vessels and works best when directed precisely at a cleanly grasped vessel. If used diffusely and to excess, as sometimes occurs after the diffuse bleeding of a heparinised cardiac reoperation, it will leave large areas of necrosis which leak serum and interfere with healing.

Topical haemostatic agents

A number of these agents have gained popularity recently and have a limited, but effective, role to play when conventional methods are not applicable. These are used for abnormal bleeding of two kinds:

(a) When blood vessels fail to retract as in the adhesions of reoperation, atheromatous vessels, porous prosthetic grafts and the vessels in solid malignant tumours. Limited retraction occurs in parenchymatous organs such as liver, spleen, kidney, thyroid and lung.

(b) In the presence of abnormal clotting due to platelet or clotting factor deficiencies, massive blood transfusion and other coagulation problems.

1   *Haemostats derived from cellulose*
Surgicel® is a knitted material made from

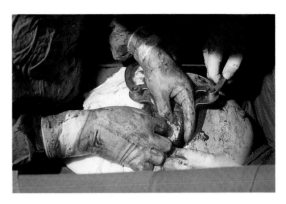

Fig 4.9 Surgicel used to stem bleeding from a penetrating wound of the lung.

polyanhydroglucoronic acid which may be particularly effective in stopping the ooze from vascular suture lines, from abnormal tissues such as tumours or from parenchymal bleeding from liver, spleen or lung when suture ligature or diathermy are ineffective. It is held in place with gentle pressure and may be left *in situ* without risk of infection or fibrosis (Fig 4.9).

2   *Fibrillary collagen*
Avitene® is a powdery, fluffy haemostat prepared from collagen. It may also be used to control capsular haemorrhage from liver, spleen or kidney. The powder is difficult to handle, sticking to gloves and instruments.

3   *Gelatin sponge with thrombin*
Gelfoam® consists of pledgets of gelatin prepared to spongelike consistency and soaked in a solution of thrombin. It is used effectively for small areas of ooze especially in neurosurgery, but has not proven useful in vascular or general surgery.

4   *Bone wax*
Beeswax is used to stop bleeding from the oozing interstices of cortical bone in cardiac and neurosurgery. Excessive use on the sternal edges may adversely affect healing of a median sternotomy.

Chapter 5

Wound Closure and Drainage

Stephen Westaby

WOUND CLOSURE

The principal aim in wound closure of traumatic or surgical wounds is to restore physical integrity and function of injured tissue without infection and with the minimum deformity. A detailed knowledge of bacteriology and the biology of wound healing, together with experience gained from treatment of war wounds during the last century, has contributed greatly to current techniques.

The method of closure selected depends on whether or not there has been tissue loss. Cleanly incised wounds, either traumatic or surgical, can be closed directly by suture whereas those with tissue deficit require skin grafts or plastic flap repair to avoid distortion. Surgical wound closure provides tissue opposition and thereby expedites haemostasis and the natural healing mechanism. The timing of wound closure is critical if a successful outcome is to be achieved. In every case a decision must be made as to whether immediate closure can be performed safely at the time of wounding or should be delayed. There are three possibilities (Fig 5.1):

Primary closure
Delayed primary closure
Healing by secondary intention.

Primary closure

This is achieved by immediate direct suture if there is no tissue loss or by plastic reconstruc-

tion with skin grafts or flap procedures if important tissue loss exists. This method is used for clean wounds without significant bacterial contamination.

Strictly, clean wounds are non traumatic, non contaminated surgical wounds where the respiratory, alimentary or genito-urinary tracts have not been entered. They are made under aseptic conditions and may be closed directly without drainage. In practice, primary closure is also applied to clean-contaminated wounds where these cavities have been entered, but without undue spread of contents and to traumatic wounds when the surgeon is satisfied that debridement or mechanical cleaning have succeeded in eliminating heavily contaminated or devitalised tissue.

Wounds contaminated by faeces, pus, infected urine or foreign material should not be closed primarily since the risks of infection and breakdown are considerable.

Delayed primary closure

In this case the wound is left open following the initial event because of significant bacterial contamination. Body cavities such as the peritoneal or pleural cavities are sealed to prevent evisceration, but drains are left *in situ*. The superficial wound layers are left open and loosely packed with dressings. Over the course of 4–5 days the wound develops resistance to infection and may then be closed by direct

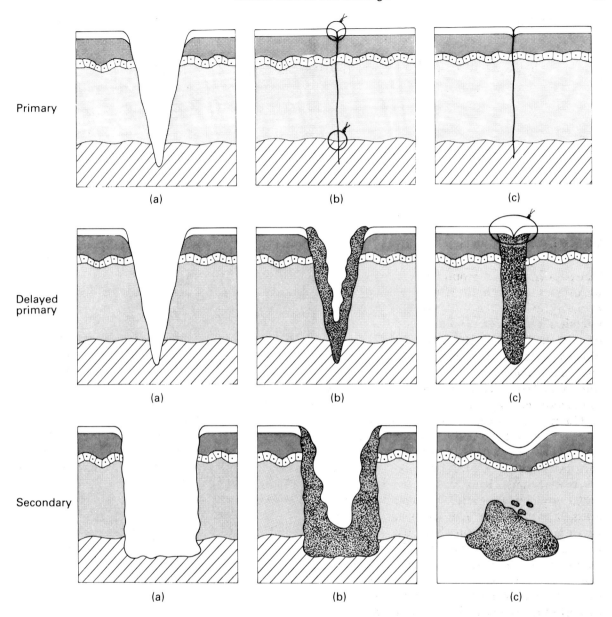

Primary

(a)   (b)   (c)

Delayed
primary

(a)   (b)   (c)

Secondary

(a)   (b)   (c)

Fig 5.1   The top row illustrates healing by primary closure; the middle row healing by delayed primary closure and the bottom row healing by secondary intention. Least scarring appears in healing by first intention.

suture or graft with only minimal risk of infection. The mechanism of this resistance has not been clearly defined, but probably depends upon the height of the inflammatory response when the leucocytes are able to combat infective organisms. The rapidity with which wounds gain resistance to infection depends on the length of time that the wound is kept open, but it is generally accepted that the optimum time for closure is on or after the 4th post-wounding day. It is notable that the presence of foreign material in a wound greatly lowers the threshold for infection. Elek showed in experiments with *Staphylococcus aureus* that the presence of a single silk suture could lower the threshold for clinical infection by a factor of 10 000. It is also apparent that wounds closed with tapes develop resistance to infection more rapidly than sutured wounds. Skin sutures actually implant small pieces of epidermis and surface organisms into deeper layers of the wound. Delayed primary closure is, therefore, best performed using a minimum of suture material, for instance by single layer mass suture of fascia and skin. When delayed closure is decided upon, the wound is covered by a sterile non-adherent dressing and not disturbed for the first 4 days unless the patient develops an unexplained fever. Unnecessary interference increases the risk of further contamination, subsequent infection and prolongation of the inflammatory phase of repair.

Healing by secondary intention

This last alternative allows the wound to close itself by a process of contraction and epithelisation. It is commonly employed for heavily contaminated or infected wounds and for extensive superficial wounds with tissue loss. The method requires careful supervision to prevent adverse scar formation, contracture and distortion, but gives good results in certain parts of the body with loose overlaying tissues such as the trunk. It is much less acceptable over underlying bone or joints where subsequent scar tissue may result in deformity. However, all wounds will eventually heal by secondary intention in the absence of an infected sinus or fistula.

This approach to the timing of wound closure is based on years of military experience with recognition that primary closure of frankly infected or heavily contaminated war wounds led to spreading infection, abscess formation, wound dehiscence, septicaemia and death. Nevertheless, inappropriate treatment of traumatic wounds still occurs in many accident departments. Indiscriminate use of modern antibiotics may compensate for this in some cases, but the combination of primary closure of a contaminated laceration with an ineffective antibiotic regime is a dangerous one. In addi-

tion to the local state of the wound, one must also consider the patient's general condition and his ability to resist infection, since the outcome of wound closure depends on many factors including his nutritional state, the integrity of the immune system and the ability to produce an inflammatory response. The local circulation must also be adequate to deliver these defence mechanisms to the site of injury.

Preparation for wound closure

Is it possible to make a contaminated wound clean, or to estimate the critical level of bacterial contamination in order to make a realistic decision as to whether to close a wound or not? In theory this should be possible and any hospital laboratory performing the routine qualitative cultures is capable of quantitative bacteriology and differentiation between normal bacterial skin flora, dangerous contamination and frank infection. Certain combinations of organisms are particularly dangerous, for instance when anaerobic organisms coexist with aerobic organisms; the latter use up the available oxygen allowing the former to flourish and multiply (e.g. *Clostridium welchii* producing gas gangrene). In practice, however, quantitative bacteriology is applied only in a few borderline clinical situations such as the timing of skin grafting for burns or pressure sores.

All traumatic wounds and some contaminated surgical wounds can be cleaned by debridement or mechanical cleaning. Debridement is considered by most surgeons to be the most important single factor in the management of the contaminated wound. This time-honoured technique has two notable aims: (a) to remove tissue contaminated by bacteria and foreign bodies, thus protecting the patient from invasive infection; (b) to remove permanently devitalised (dead or ischaemic) tissue.

All foreign matter or devitalised soft tissue left in a wound damages its defence against infection. Dead fat, muscle and skin act as a culture medium promoting bacterial growth and also inhibit white cell migration and phagocytosis of invading organisms.

Scalpel, scissors, forceps and the surgeon's time are much more effective in this procedure than enzymes and dressing regimens. A general anaesthetic is almost always required, since radical excision of unwanted tissue must be performed. Identification of the limits of devitalised tissue in a wound is difficult especially in the case of muscle. Colour, consistency and the ability to bleed are reasonable guides, but perhaps the best is the ability of the muscle to contract when stimulated by the cutting blade. Skin is easier to assess especially after 24 hours when a sharp line of demarcation usually exists between dead and viable skin.

When a heavily contaminated wound contains specialised tissue, such as nerves or tendons, complete excision is not feasible. In such cases high pressure irrigation followed by excision of all fragments that are not clearly viable is indicated.

A specific exception to the general principle of removing all devitalised tissue is made in treating specialised tissues that perform an important physical function regardless of viability. Tissues like dura, fascia and tendon may survive as free grafts without living cells if immediately covered by healthy pedicle flaps. Cells from the wound may then invade the graft as part of the healing process. If these tissues can be rendered surgically clean they should be left in the wound.

Mechanical cleansing

This has two goals – removal of noxious substances from the wound and protection of wound healing mechanisms by providing an optimal local environment. The two basic methods employed to cleanse a wound are hydraulic force and direct contact.

Perhaps the most useful manoeuvre in topical wound care is irrigation. The hydraulic pressure of an irrigating stream of fluid dislodges contaminants and serves to reduce bacterial colonisation. Interestingly, it takes smaller hydraulic forces to rid the wound of large foreign bodies than it does to remove bacteria. High pressure irrigation has been shown to be effective in removing bacteria from wounds, but concern that high pressure can damage tissue defences seems justified.

Pulsitile high pressure syringe irrigation results in trauma to the tissues that makes the wound more susceptible to experimental infection. Low pressure irrigation, with a bulb syringe, is less effective in removing bacteria, but is also less damaging to the tissues. The author compromises by using a high volume rapid flow system with weak antiseptic solutions through a wound irrigation device which allows irrigation of contaminated wounds with a closed system of drainage (Fig 5.2).

Another method often employed to cleanse a wound is direct mechanical contact by scrubbing the dirty wound with a sponge. This cannot be accomplished without anaesthesia, but is an effective means of removing bacteria. Unfortunately, despite this benefit, scrubbing the wound with a saline soaked sponge does not decrease the incidence of infection.

Tissue trauma inflicted by the sponge impairs the wound's ability to resist infection and allows the residual bacteria to elicit an inflammatory response. The addition of a nontoxic surfactant such as Pleuronic Polyol F68 minimises tissue damage while maintaining the

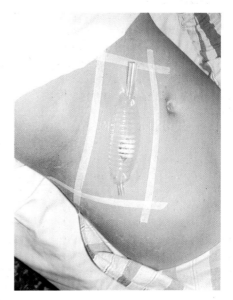

Fig 5.2 Wound irrigation device. (Squibb Surgicare Ltd.)

efficiency of mechanical cleansing. Consequently, use of a surfactant soaked sponge reduces the incidence of infection in contaminated wounds in experimental animals.

Aspects of suture technique in primary wound closure

From a technical standpoint there are three vital factors in suture technique. They are the tightness of the suture tie, the size of the tissue bite and the distance between sutures. In 1938 Whipple commented that 'tight suturing is probably the commonest mistake made in the repair of abdominal incisions'. His research showed microscopic evidence of necrosis under tightly tied sutures (Fig 5.3).

In one of the few published experimental studies of tightly tied sutures, Nelson found the 7 day tensile strength of wounds closed with tight ties to be 48% of normal compared with 63% for wounds closed with loose ties and microscopic studies showed tissue necrosis around tightly tied sutures. This necrosis leads to weaker wounds more susceptible to rupture under increased intra-abdominal pressure. A loose tie is one that provides just enough tension to permit the fascial edges to touch. There should be no wrinkling of the fascia.

Larger bites of tissue within the suture result in stronger wounds than small bites. This is probably because they are more resistant to cutting through the tissue than small bites. It has been shown experimentally that small bites

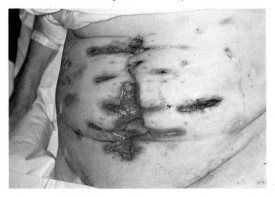

Fig 5.3 Wound dehiscence resulting from excessively tight suturing.

tear through the tissues, especially if tied too tightly and this certainly predisposes to wound dehiscence.

In another experiment Nelson found that increasing the distance between sutures from 1 to 2 cm doubled the strength of sutured abdominal wounds and by increasing the number of sutures no additional strength could be gained. Also when compared to closure by simple interrupted suture, wounds closed with continuous suture techniques show more extensive and prolonged oedema and induration and more sluggish circulation.

It has been shown that at 2 weeks after wound closure the burst strength of a wound closed with continuous suture is markedly less than a similar wound closed by interrupted sutures. It is possible that the swelling and mirocirculatory effects both affect collagen synthesis and result in prolongation of the destructive, inflammatory phase of healing and delay the onset of that phase during which collagen synthesis can contribute significantly to the strength of the wound (Fig 5.4). A continuous suture can be conceptualised as a single element helical coil fixed at both ends and filled with tissue. As the tissue swells in response to injury, tension is placed on the suture and the intervening circulation is compromised. The suture then cuts into the tissues and if skin is sutured in this manner the unsightly cross hatching of the scar results.

The correct choice of suture materials can be critical. There are both advantages and disadvantages in each type of suture material which renders it uniquely good, or bad, in part — or all — of a wound in a specific anatomic area under specific clinical circumstances. Size and tensile strength of the sutures must be matched to the holding strength of the tissue in which they are placed. Measurement of the *in vivo* degradation of sutures separates them into two general classes.

Sutures that rapidly undergo degradation in tissue, losing their tensile strength within 60 days, can be considered *absorbable* sutures. Those which maintain their tensile strength for longer than 60 days after implantation may be

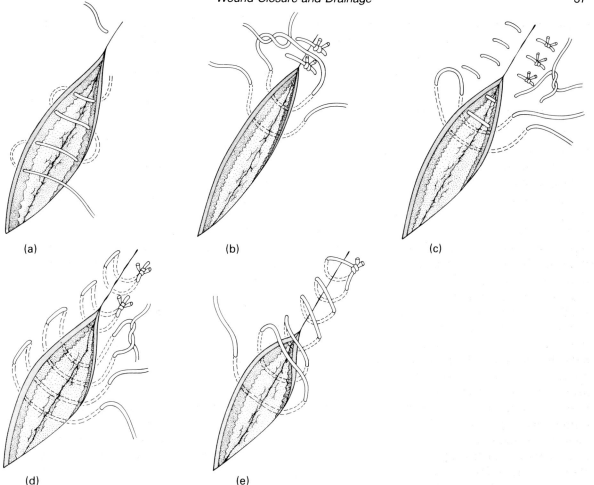

Fig 5.4 Sutures and tying techniques. (a) Subcuticular suture; (b) Interrupted over-and-over suture; (c) Interrupted vertical mattress suture; (d) Interrupted horizontal mattress suture; (e) Continuous over-and-over suture.

referred to as *non-absorbable*. In practice, this terminology is misleading since some so called non-absorbable sutures, such as silk, cotton and nylon, lose their tensile strength rapidly after the 2nd month and by the 6th month have either disintegrated or are so weak that they have little or no effect in reinforcing the tissue.

The absorbable sutures are gut, derived from sheep submucosa or beef serosa, and the synthetics, polyglycolic acid and polyglactin. Treatment of gut with chromium salts, a cross linking agent, prolongs retention of the suture's tensile strength and increases its resistance to absorbtion by enzyme action. Suture materials are considered in greater depth in Chapter 6.

Skin wounds are subject to considerably less stress than fascial wounds and need support for only short periods of time. If percutaneous sutures are employed, early removal before the 7th postwounding day should be instituted before epithelisation of the suture track occurs.

It is well known that the incidence of infection in contaminated wounds, approximated by even the least reactive suture, is significantly higher than similar wounds closed by tapes. This, together with the superior cosmetic results and better patient acceptability, has influenced the author to use methods of sutureless skin closure over the past few years (Figs 5.5a, 5.5b).

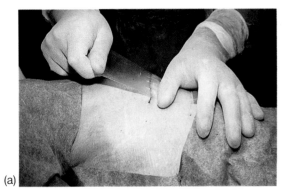

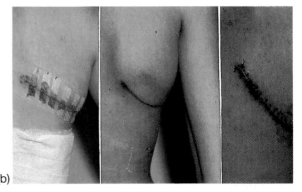

(a)   (b)

Fig 5.5 (a) Op-site® sutureless skin closure. (b) Three different methods of closure of pleurectomy wound (lateral thoracotomy).

The ease with which wounds can be closed by tape varies considerably according to the anatomic and biomechanical properties of the wound site. The relatively lax skin of the face and abdomen makes it amenable to wound closure by tapes. In contrast, the taut skin of the extremities, subject to frequent dynamic joint movements, limits the adherence of most tape and the success of closure.

The copious secretions from the skin of the axillae, palms and soles also discourage tape adherence. Of course, some wounds, such as lacerations resulting from impact injuries — when closing the wound is like putting together a jigsaw puzzle — demand careful suture closure to obtain a cosmetic result.

Under these circumstances, fine monofilament, non-absorbable synthetic sutures are best. Sutures which provide an intense inflammatory reaction (silk and cotton) should be avoided at all costs. Tape closure is probably good for sharp lacerations where the wound edges can be accurately approximated. The bonus of this technique is that children are spared painful injections of local anaesthetic required for suturing.

Metal clips have been used for closure of skin wounds for many years (Fig 5.6). Their only advantage is speed of application and it has been shown by Harrison that wounds closed with clips are significantly weaker and have a lower modulus of elasticity. Recent experiments have shown stapled skin wounds to be more susceptible to infection than taped wounds.

There have been a number of interesting developments in the field of tissue adhesives such as cyanocrylate in the repair of organs and haemostatic agents in emergency or mass combat casualty situations. There is evidence, however, that their use should not include skin closure. While adhesives have been used to bond skin wounds, the polymers used act as a barrier between the growing edges of the wound. This delays healing and histotoxic reactions in the wounded tissue again predispose to infection.

In practice, primary closure is best per-

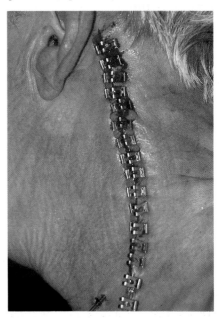

Fig 5.6 Clipped wound.

formed with the minimum of suture material and with careful attention to suture technique. Skin sutures should be avoided whenever possible, using tape closure to maintain apposition of the skin edges.

Complications after surgical wound closure

Besides wound infection there are three principal complications after primary wound closure. These are wound dehiscence (Figs 5.7: 5.8), incisional hernia and wound sinus formation, all of which are seen most frequently following abdominal operations. After laparotomy, complete wound dehiscence leads to burst abdomen and evisceration of bowel which is both a frightening and dangerous complication for the patient. Incisional hernia occurs when the muscle and fascial layers give way, but the skin remains intact. Though this situation may be apparent before the patient leaves hospital, an incisional hernia enlarges progressively to the point of inconvenience. Sinus formation usually occurs when underlying suture material becomes infected and a small abscess tracks to the wound surface and discharges pus. In the presence of foreign mate-

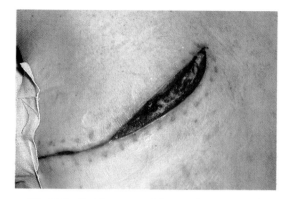

Fig 5.8 Dehiscence of thoracotomy wound.

rial the discharge becomes chronic and though antibiotics may give temporary relief, the sinus will persist until the foreign material is removed.

Both local and systemic factors predispose to these complications. Local factors include suture technique and the materials used, precision of apposition of the wound edges and the integrity of blood supply to the area. Wound dehiscence occurs if the sutures are unable to hold the wound edges together until the wound has acquired sufficient strength of its own through the healing process. This can be due to:

a premature reduction of the strength of the suture material;
b insufficient strength of the thread itself in the tied suture loop;
c cutting of the suture through its opposed tissues.

Wound drains should be brought out through a separate incision and not the wound itself. Absorbable sutures such as catgut and polyglyconic acid (Dexon) have a much higher wound failure rate than non-absorbable sutures such as nylon after laparotomy and should be avoided in this situation.

Wound infection is by far the most important single factor associated with failure and was found to be the underlying cause in 48% of burst abdomens and 85% of wound sinuses in a recent survey of laparotomies. The aetiology of incisional hernia and burst abdomen are simi-

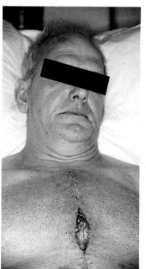
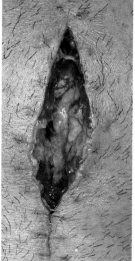

Fig 5.7 Dehiscence of median sternotomy after cardiac surgery.

lar and multifactorial. They include old age, male sex, obesity, abdominal distension and postoperative chest infection with coughing. Both are most common after bowel surgery.

General factors influencing the frequency of postoperative wound complications are those which result in poor healing and include jaundice, diabetes and malignant diseases.

Bucknall at the Westminster Hospital in London studied 1129 laparotomy wounds after a 5-year period and found overall 19 burst abdomens (1.68%), 84 incisional herniae (7.44%) and 76 wound sinuses (6.73%). Part way through this study the surgeons changed technique from suture of each individual layer of the wound to the mass closure method which originated at the Cleveland Clinic.

Mass closure involves suture of all layers apart from the subcutaneous fat and skin using wide bites at least 1 cm away from the edge of the incision. The comparative incidence of burst abdomen for the two methods using nylon suture were:

Mass closure
  788 patients with 6 dehiscences (0.76%)
Individual layer closure
  341 patients with 13 dehiscences (3.81%)

It seems clear, therefore, that the mass suture technique is preferable to multilayered closure. When mass closure with nylon was compared with mass closure with polyglycolic acid the failure rate (overall complications) was 4.7% as compared with 12.5%. It was felt that the rate of sinus formation would be lower with the absorbable material, but this was not the case (9.5% with nylon, 11.5% with polyglycolic acid). One hypothesis to account for this is that bacteria hide in the braid and knots of suture material. Non-braided material may, therefore, be preferable. Moynihan's statement (1920) that 'Every operation in surgery is an experiment in bacteriology' remains true today.

WOUND DRAINAGE

'When in doubt, drain'
  — Lawsen Tait, 1845–99.

Tait was an eminent English surgeon who made many original contributions in both general and gynaecological surgery. In his time many elective operations carried a prohibitive mortality through sepsis. Drainage tubes which allowed pus to escape from the abdomen or chest were life-saving in the pre-antibiotic era and their omission was considered negligent.

Development and refinement of aseptic technique, better methods of sterilisation and the principles of wound debridement and delayed primary closure allowed Lord Moynihan to state that 'drainage of the peritoneal cavity is rarely necessary' even before the introduction of antibiotics as we know them. Though knowledge of the use or misuse and dangers of drainage has increased since that time, there is no uniformity in its application. Every surgeon has his own indications and methods, and will fiercely disagree with others.

Drainage may be used either as a method of treatment or to prevent complications. It may be therapeutic or prophylactic.

Therapeutic drainage

An abscess is an enclosed collection of pus which results from an acute inflammatory reaction in response to local infection. Pus consists of serum, dead white cells and bacteria, some live bacteria and necrotic tissue debris from the affected tissue. Chemical degradation products released into the surrounding hyperaemic circulation and the accompanying bacteraemia or septicaemia result in an unpleasant systemic illness with fever, rigors, sweating, dehydration, loss of appetite and depression. Abscesses may be found in any part of the body and cannot be sterilised or cured by antibiotics alone. Surgical drainage is required to relieve both local and systemic symptoms. Common sites of abscess formation are listed in Table 1.

Each has in common a closed tissue space or part of a body cavity where pus accumulates under pressure. Progressive enlargement of an abscess may give rise to disturbances of vital structures as in the case of cerebral abscess

Table 1
COMMON SITES OF ABCESS FORMATION

Skin	Boil, furuncle or carbuncle
Appendix	Appendix abscess
Gallbladder	Empyema of the gallbladder
Liver	Liver abscess
Pelvis of kidney	Pyonephrosis
Peritoneal cavity	Pelvic subphrenic or paracolic abscess
Pericardium	Purulent pericarditis
Pleural cavity	Empyema
Lung	Lung abscess
Brain	Cerebral abscess
Labia	Bartholins abscess
Fallopian tube	Pyosalpinx
Surgical wound	Wound abscess

where the rigid cranial cavity limits expansion or purulent pericarditis where the fluid causes cardiac tamponade. Surgical drainage with placement of tube drains proves life-saving. Therapeutic drainage may also be required in the treatment of extravasations of bile or pancreatic juice in the peritoneal cavity. It was common in the past to employ stab suprapubic drainage or even multiple site drainage of the peritoneal cavity for all forms of diffuse peritonitis. However, it is now understood that much of the peritoneal exudate is protective, so this practice has been largely discontinued. Drainage in diffuse peritonitis is placed only to an area where abscess formation has become established.

Prophylactic drainage

This is required wherever physiological fluid is expected to collect after a surgical procedure or when an anastomosis or closure of a viscus could leak. For example, bile may escape after operations on the bile ducts or liver; pancreatice juice after operations on the pancreas and urine after operations on, or injuries to, the kidney. Different surgeons differ widely in their attitudes and approach to the necessity for prophylactic drainage since drainage itself may lead to problems.

Some consider it wise to employ drainage if it is feared than intestinal secretions may escape following intestinal strangulation or injury, or operations on the bowel (for example colectomy in obese, infected or frail patients.) Drainage in the neighbourhood of the duodenal stump after gastrectomy is advisable if the closure is unavoidably unsatisfactory, although drainage is no substitute for poor surgical technique.

After evacuation of certain cysts, it may be advisable to insert a drain in order to prevent reformation of the cyst. An example is the pancreatic pseudocyst, although internal drainage by anastomosis of the cyst to the stomach may be preferred. Formerly drainage was routinely employed for hydatid cysts of the liver. Nowadays, it is more customary to fill the cyst with saline, then close the liver. The cyst will disappear slowly as the saline is absorbed. Drainage is also used to deflect natural body fluids along an alternative route in order to 'rest' a new suture line, as in T-tube drainage of the common bile duct and urinary diversion via a nephrostomy or suprapubic catheter after surgery in the urinary tract.

One of the most common reasons for drainage is when haemostasis has been difficult to achieve during an operation. This occurs, for example, after hepatic lobectomy, splenectomy, fractured pelvis or pelvic eventertion, pleural decortication or cardiac surgery when the patient has been heparinised. Here there is a second objective – the diagnosis of secondary or reactive haemorrhage when a drain to the surgical site provides rapid evidence of impending problems.

A wound in which good haemostasis has not been secured should be drained to prevent haematoma formation with the risk of wound breakdown. In this instance, closed vacuum drainage is useful in order to minimise the risk of wound infection entering along the drainage track. Vacuum drainage of extensive raw surfaces is advisable when haematoma formation may prejudice healing of the overlying skin flaps as in mastectomy, limb amputation or plastic reconstructive procedures over the chest, back or abdomen (Fig 5.9).

Drainage of the deep layers of an abdominal

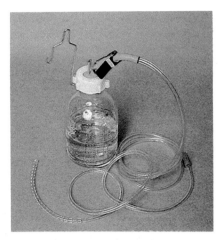

Fig 5.9 Vacuum drain.

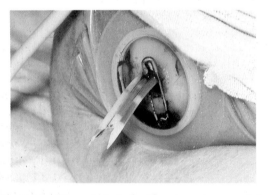

Fig 5.10 Wound drain to the deep layers of the abdominal wall after appendicectomy.

wound rather than the peritoneal cavity may be desireable on occasions, for example when the wound is contaminated by pus after drainage of an appendix abscess or empyema of the gallbladder (Fig 5.10).

Most intraperitoneal abscesses tend to point towards a previous abdominal incision and, therefore, some surgeons, when dealing with cases where it is feared an abdominal abscess may arise, put a drain down to, but not through, the closed peritoneum. This directs and facilitates the passage of pus through the more superficial layers of the wound.

Principles of peritoneal drainage

In therapeutic drainage the pus should be drained whenever possible by the shortest route from the abscess to the skin surface to avoid opening the peritoneal cavity. In prophylactic drainage the drain should be placed down to the site where fluid is expected to collect; good positioning is important. Intraperitoneal collections tend to escape to where they find a way out of the general peritoneal cavity. Such collections have a strong tendency to find their way towards recent operative incisions or even to old scars or sites of previous peritoneal drainage. If no such scar is present, they track to the umbilicus.

Pelvic abscesses tend to point and burst through the rectum or posterior vault of the vagina, or into the bladder before they point on the abdominal wall. Abscesses around the gallbladder tend to burst into neighbouring organs such as the colon or duodenum, before they approach the skin.

The main object of drainage is to establish a track along which secretions can escape to the exterior rather than finding their own way. Ideally, this track should follow the natural, preferential drainage track, but this is not always practical. If the incision is placed in such a position that gravity helps the drainage, the abscess cavity will tend to remain empty and consequently its walls will come together with more rapid healing.

In draining an appendix abscess, the incision should be over the tender or indurated area, preferably well over to the right side away from the small bowel. Every endeavour should be made to dissect extraperitoneally and to open the abscess without opening the peritoneal cavity. The abscess region is tentatively explored with a finger with suction held nearby. The moment pus is detected suction is applied to the cavity which is aspirated dry. A tube drain (or corrugated latex, or Penrose drain) is then introduced and ideally brought to the surface through the nearest point to the skin, if necessary by a separate stab wound.

Drainage is also employed in closing the wound itself, a soft, fine rubber tube being placed down to the closed peritoneum. As an alternative, delayed primary closure may be employed, leaving the wound packed open for 3 days until the major risk of infection by contamination has passed. After 48 hours, bowel and omentum are so well matted around an intraperitoneal drain that a good drainage track has formed and the side holes of the tube drain are closed off. Consequently, the drain may be shortened perhaps by 3–5 cm each day, aiming to have it completely removed within 4–15 days of operation.

Principles of chest drainage

A chest tube is simply a drain like any other drain, and is used to remove air, blood or pus from the pleural cavity, preventing compression of the lung or allowing it to re-expand. Besides draining air and fluid out of the pleural space, a chest drainage system must also prevent their return, encouraged by the negative intrapleural pressure created by breathing in. For this dual job three components are required:

1 An unobstructed chest tube of adequate diameter.
2 A collecting container below the chest level.
3 A one-way mechanism — a water seal or Heimlich valve to prevent the return of air or fluid.

A patient may have one or two tubes inserted, or occasionally more, depending on the kind of drainage present. Because air rises and liquid sinks, the tip placed to drain air is in the apex of the pleural space and that for liquid at the base posterolaterally in the costophrenic angle. The chest tube will be joined to about 1.8m of connecting tubing which leads to a bottle placed several feet below the patient's chest. This tubing allows him to turn and move and minimises the chance that a deep breath could suck liquid back into his chest.

The position of the bottle and underwater seal takes advantage of gravity flow by establishing the patient's pleural space as the area of higher pressure and the collecting bottle as the area of lower pressure. The non-patient end of the tubing is led below the surface of sterile water which serves to create a 'water seal' and

to establish a closed system by sealing off the open end of the tubing from the atmosphere (Fig 5.11). The positive pressure in the chest during exhalation can push air and liquid out of the pleural cavity. The air bubbles out through the water and out of the vent tube of the drainage bottle while liquid mixes with the water. The length of tube drain below the water surface should be short so that the resistance to air escape is no more than 2–3 cm of water pressure. If, for instance, the drainage bottle was full of liquid (say blood from chest trauma) then the resistance to air passage through the underwater part of the tube (say 15–20 cm of water) could prevent air escape and produce a pneumothorax even in the presence of a 'functioning chest drain'.

A traditional procedure that constitutes a life-threatening hazard is the practice of clamping a chest tube on the slightest pretext that the drainage bottle might be upset or broken (to that end two haemostats with rubber tubing over their tip are commonly kept within instant reach). Note that any time the tube is clamped, no air or liquid can escape from the pleural space and this puts the patient with a pleural air leak in real danger of developing a tension pneumothorax. A pneumothorax can take two

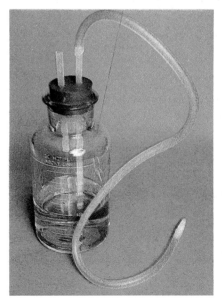

Fig 5.11 Underwater seal drain.

forms — open and closed. If a chest tube becomes disconnected, thus opening the pleural cavity to the atmosphere, the lung collapses away from the chest wall by a relatively small amount and its ventilation is impaired since it no longer expands efficiently. As long as the hole in the chest wall is smaller than the trachea, however, an open pneumothorax is well tolerated since the other lung continues to function normally.

By contrast, if the chest tube is clamped in a patient with an air leak from the surface of the lung, air enters the pleural space, but cannot get out. Each time the patient breathes in, more air escapes, builds up in the pleural cavity and compresses the lung. Sometimes, the pressure builds up rapidly and the lung collapses totally, the mediastinum is pushed over to the opposite side and then the opposite lung is also compressed. This is a tension pneumothorax. Compression of the mediastinum by air under pressure interferes with venous return to the heart and reduces cardiac output. Eventually, impairment of ventilation and reduced cardiac output cause death.

It is appropriate *never* to clamp chest tubes, either when the patient gets out of bed, walks, or is taken to some other part of the hospital or, indeed, is transferred from one hospital to another. Every thoracic surgical unit has seen patients who have died during transfer from a general hospital and who have had their chest drains clamped.

The bottle should be handled carefully, as one would any piece of equipment attached to a patient, and kept below chest level, making sure the water seal is intact. If the drainage tubing comes loose from the bottles, the end must be cleaned, reconnected and the patient should be asked calmly to cough a few times. This will rid the pleural cavity of most of the pneumothorax. For a patient who has never had an air leak, clamping for a short time·when changing the drainage bottles does no harm. It is just so much better to be in the 'no clamping' than clamping habit.

Drains to the pericardium or mediastinum after cardiac surgery do not usually communicate with the pleural cavity and need not drain to an underwater seal. However, when the diaphragm has been opened and only partially closed — for instance in resection of carcinoma of the stomach and oesophagus — any drain left to the upper abdomen should be of the water seal type to prevent development of a pneumothorax.

Disadvantages of drainage

Drains act as retrograde conduits through which skin contaminants gain entrance to the wound and the presence of the drain itself impairs the resistance of tissues to infection. This effect can be minimised by using a closed system of drainage with as few connections as possible (for example, Redi-Vac® with vacuum bottle as compared to a corrugated drain opening into dressings).

Abdominal drains have been shown to impair wound healing and healing in intestinal anastomoses. Though the exact mechanism of the effect is unknown, it is obvious that drains are foreign bodies and that they prevent the collapse of normal tissues against the anastomosis. The retrograde conduction of bacteria may contaminate the dead space caused by the drain at the anastomotic site, thereby predisposing to infection and leakage.

If the drain impinges directly on a blood vessel or viscus, this may produce pressure necrosis with fistula formation or secondary haemorrhage. These risks may be eliminated initially by correct siting of the drain, by only using soft rubber materials, and by shortening the drain at intervals so that it does not remain in contact with any single structure for more than 48 hours.

Unfortunately, when a drain is used prophylactically against dehiscence of a bowel or gastric anastomosis, this may not occur until after the 5th postoperative day. If a drain is left in place for too long, the intestine may become kinked and obstructed by becoming either adherent or involved in adhesions forming around it.

Drains brought out through the original

abdominal incision produce a source of weakness in the scar that may eventually lead to the development of an incisional hernia. Drains should, therefore, whenever possible, be brought out through a separate stab incision and great care should be taken not to damage the epigastric vessels in the rectus sheath (anterior abdominal wall).

When to remove the drain

When a drain no longer performs the function for which it was intended, it should be removed immediately even if this is within a few hours of operation. A drain that fails to function is a constant source of danger. General guidelines for removal of a drain are as follows:

1 When drainage has stopped; for instance an air leak or blood loss after chest trauma, bleeding from mediastinal drains after cardiac surgery or bile drainage that may occur after liver trauma or cholecystectomy.
2 When an abscess cavity has closed. This may be easy to determine for superficial abscesses, but inaccessible cavities such as thoracic collections may need repeated instillation of contrast medium and x-ray to follow their progress.
3 When repair is complete as after T-tube drainage of the common bile duct after its exploration.
4 When there is a risk of drain-related complications. Some patients with a prolonged air leak after lung resection require intercostal drainage for as long as 2 to 3 weeks. Pressure of the tube drain on intercostal vessels under the rib then gives rise to a significant risk of erosion and major haemorrhage. This must be avoided by changing the position of the drain.

Materials used for drainage tubes

Ideally these materials should be non-irritant to the tissues. Red rubber used to be the most popular material – it is soft, pliable, easy to sterilise and produces minimal pressure on adjacent structures. However, it evokes an irritant reaction and has been replaced by latex rubber. Silicone rubber is even less irritant. It is also soft and pliable, but expensive.

Drains made of plastic materials such a polyvinyl chloride are inert in the tissues and do not become as easily infected as rubber. Many of these materials lose their pliability when sterilised and may become rigid in the body and produce pressure damage. A radiopaque strip is a useful addition to modern drains.

Types of drain

Pauls tubing

This strip of rubber, useful for draining subcutaneous tissue, has now been largely superceded by Redi-Vac drains.

Corrugated strips of rubber or plastic

These are still used to drain the fat layers and subcutaneous tissues of a contaminated wound and, by some, to drain the peritoneal cavity where tube drains may produce pressure necrosis (Fig 5.12). They drain into surface dressings, are messy and produce a conduit for access of bacteria when the dressings are removed.

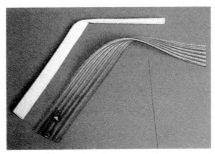

Fig 5.12 Penrose drain (*top*); corrugated drain (*bottom*).

Tubes and catheters

These are the most efficient type of drain for escape of pus or fluid and are used almost exclusively for chest drainage. It is best to connect a tube drain to a closed drainage bag below the level of the wound so that flow is aided by gravity. Access of organisms through the drain is eliminated, although if the tube is inadequately fixed, the skin movement at this point will encourage infection around the drain site.

The intracavity part of the drain may be cut to provide channels or drainage holes to facilitate passage of fluids. When holes are cut they should be small so that intestine cannot invaginate itself into the drain and kink. Drainage into dressings is unsatisfactory since dressings obstruct the lumen, rapidly become offensive, provide a portal of entry for bacteria and do not allow accurate measurement of escaping material.

Suction may be applied to tube drains and provides a more efficient method of assisted drainage than obliteration of 'dead space' by pressure (as in pressure dressings after mastectomy).

'Sump drains' were popular for draining large quantities of fluid from a deep wound or fistula in the peritoneal cavity. The sump is constructed from a tube of either rubber, plastic or stainless steel with holes in its wall to allow fluid to enter and collect in its lumen. The fluid can then be removed by suction through a rubber catheter connected to a vacuum pump. Recently, it has been shown that suction increases the risks of infection by drawing bacteria into the wound and that the likelihood of infection increases with increasing suction pressure.

The most popular suction drainage system at present is the closed Redi-Vac system where suction is provided by negative pressure from a bottle. This is ideal for removal of blood and serous fluid from superficial wounds and incisions without significant increase in the risk of infection. When negative pressure is low and suction is inadequate for drainage, a new bottle is substituted.

Wick drains

These function by the same principle as the oil lamp where oil travels up a wick, against gravity, by capillary action. The Penrose drain is the most popular variety and is widely used in the United States (Fig 5.12). This consists of a tube of soft latex which contains a gauze wick. It is soft and malleable and, therefore, does not cause pressure necrosis. It is also non-irritant to the tissues and can be safely left in the peritoneal cavity for a week.

Chapter 6

Sutures in Wound Repair

Ian Capperauld

INTRODUCTION

Often the choice of suture material is an emotional and not a scientific decision, based on what the surgeon has been taught by his Chief. Over the past 30 years there has been a tremendous increase in the types of suture material available, especially with the introduction of man made fibres. There are relatively few papers in the surgical journals concerning suture materials and often the data obtainable from the manufacturers is scanty in its technical details. Papers written 30 or 40 years ago on suture materials are now totally inaccurate since manufacturing changes of well established suture materials have improved them considerably. Surgical technique is far more important than the suture material used, but a good working knowledge of the properties of the various suture materials available will ensure a choice based more on fact than on fiction.

The purpose of a suture is to hold a wound together in good apposition until such time as the natural wound healing process is sufficiently well established to make the support from the suture material unnecessary and redundant. There are four key words in this statement, namely, *Hold*, *Apposition*, *Wound Healing* and *Redundant*. If each of these key words is expanded in the context of suture contribution, this will serve as a base line to a discussion on individual suture materials.

Hold

Wounds break down following a surgical procedure for many reasons. Most of these are non suture related and are due to haematoma formation, infection, paralytic ileus and rise in pressure from violent coughing and sneezing. However, the following list represents the causes of wound breakdown which could be suture related.

1 *The suture breaks*; probably because too small a size has been used.
2 *The suture cuts out*; due to too fine a material having been used with friable tissue or too much tension having been placed on the suture.
3 *The knot slips*; due to inadequate tying of the knot which will be described later in the chapter.
4 *The suture is extruded*; in combination with infection of the wound either early or late.
5 *The suture absorbs too rapidly*; when an absorbable suture has been put into a situation where a non-absorbable should have been used.
6 *The suture has been removed too early*; when the support given by the suture is still necessary for the stage of healing that the wound has reached.

Table 1 shows the result of an experiment where the suture pull-out value of tissues has

Table 1

Tissue	Suture pull and value in pounds (kg)	
Fat	0.44	(0.20)
Peritoneum	1.9	(0.86)
Muscle	2.8	(1.27)
Fascia	8.3	(3.77)

been calculated by placing a loop of suture material into a particular tissue and then applying a measured force until that suture pulls out of the tissue. This value, expressed in lbs or kilos represents the holding capacity of that particular tissue.

Table 2 shows the nearest size of suture material which has a breaking strain the same as or similar to the suture pull-out value and from this the selection of the suitable size of suture material related to the tissue can be made. In practice, surgeons generally tend to use too thick a size of suture material for the particular tissues in which they are working. The thicker the suture material the larger the foreign body and this is compounded when knotted, as the knot represents an even larger foreign body.

degree of apposition is undertaken with the tissues beneath the skin and this is extremely important to obtain good healing. The following points, therefore, should be noted when placing the sutures to get the best apposition.

1 The various layers should be apposed accurately.
2 The knots should be tied with minimum tension to avoid strangulation.
3 Minimum trauma must be used when the sutures are implanted.
4 The finest practical suture size should be chosen.
5 The correct knot should be tied to ensure it will not slip.
6 The correct suture length should be used.

In general, the length of suture used to close an incision should be four times the length of that incision. This can be achieved by taking big bites away from the edge of the wound where there is liable to be a collagenolytic effect occasioned by the trauma of the implantation for a distance of approximately 5 mm from the edge of the wound.

Healing

A description of wound healing is given in

Table 2

Tissue	Suture pull-out value (kg)	B.S. in kg & size Catgut		B.S. in kg & size silk	
Fat	0.2	0.31	6/0	0.20	7/0
Peritoneum	0.86	1.5	5/0	0.82	5/0
Muscle	1.27	1.70	4/0	1.70	4/0
Fascia	3.77	3.70	2/0	3.70	2/0

Apposition

During most surgical procedures, great care is taken on closing the skin to ensure that the edges are accurately apposed, that there is no dog earing and no overlapping. The reasons for this are many, but not the least of which is that this is the show-piece of the surgeon's skill and that which is visible to the patient and the relatives. However, frequently not the same

Chapter 3. However, it should be remembered that different tissues heal at varying rates. Figure 6.1 shows the variation between tissues such as skin, colon, stomach and the urinary bladder.

It will be apparent, therefore, that one could choose a suture material with tensile strength loss which would match the tensile strength gain of the wound to ensure that when the

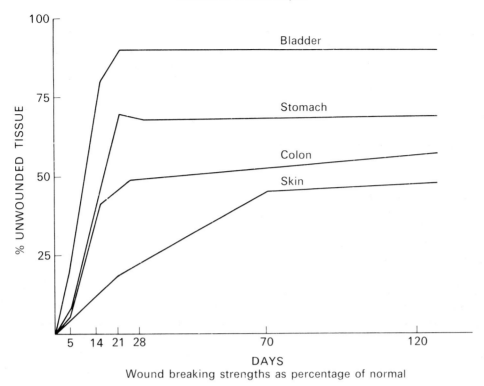

Fig 6.1 Comparison in rate of wound healing for different tissues.

redundancy of the suture occurs, it will be at the optimal time. This can be expressed in a formula:

The total strength = the instrinsic strength
of a wound (the wound healing)
+ the extrinsic strength
(the contribution made
by the suture).

The tissue which takes the longest time to heal is fascia which has only regained 75% of its original tensile strength at 280 days.

Redundant

The ideal situation in a healing wound would be for the suture material to disappear completely once its extrinsic role in wound support has been completed. However, the present state of knowledge of suture manufacturers and polymer chemists is such that this ideal state has not yet been reached, but with advances in polymer technology it could well be that the future will see materials with tensile strength loss and absorption profiles which will accurately match the particular tissue requirements. However, remaining suture materials, having completed their object, are redundant for the following reasons:

1 The suture is a foreign body.
2 It could be the site for latent infection with subsequent herniation or extrusion.
3 It could be the site for stone formation, e.g., in the cystic duct following cholecystectomy or in the urinary bladder following an intravesical procedure.
4 It could form the site for an anastomotic ulcer in gastrointestinal anastomosis or in colonic anastomosis.

SUTURE MATERIALS

Before discussing individual suture materials there are many ways of classifying them and Table 3 will help to form a basis of understanding of the various differences.

By using the above classifications it will be apparent that a suture material could be described more accurately using this knowledge. Thus, silk is of biological origin coming from the cocoon of the silk worm; it is braided; it is coated with wax to reduce capillarity and to make it stiffer; and it is non-absorbable. In contrast, polydioxanone is a man-made or synthetic material, monofilament, uncoated and absorbable.

Main properties of suture materials

There are seven main properties in suture materials which aid the surgeon in making the appropriate selection of material related to the particular operative procedure which he is undertaking. These properties are listed below.

Size

Up until a few years ago one of the areas of confusion was the sizing of suture materials. This is not surprising when a fibre of 0.008 – 0.1

inches was called a No. 3 nylon; a No. 36 or 40 cotton; a No. 80 linen; a No. 2/0 or 1/0 Pearsall's Chinese twisted silk; a No. 1 Pearsall's braided silk; a 33 SWG wire; 3/0 boilable Catgut or 4/0 non-boilable Catgut. However, both an imperial and metric system have now been introduced which is approved by both the United States Pharmacopoeia and the European Pharmacopoeia. Table 4 shows the accepted sizing of sutures by diameter. There is a slight variation in diameter for non-absorbables when compared to absorbables since these figures were drawn up when the only absorbable was Catgut which, on wetting, became swollen and therefore had a higher diameter for its size.

Tensile strength

The tensile strength of suture materials is controlled by the United States Pharmacopoeia and the European Pharmacopoeia. Tensile strength is defined as the load applied per unit of cross sectional area and is quoted in psi or kg/cm^2. In practice, however, it is usually the breaking strength of materials which is considered and this is defined as the force required to break a suture regardless of its diameter and is quoted in 1b or kg. When dealing with suture materials, both the straight and the knot pull strength are considered, the latter being in

Table 3

Absorbable	*Non-absorbable*
Catgut, collagen, homopolymer of glycolide, copolymers of glycolide and lactide, homopolymer of polydioxanone	Polyester, polyamide, polypropylene, polyethylene, steel, silk, cotton, linen
Biological	*Man-made*
Catgut, collagen, silk, linen, cotton	Polyester, polyamide, polypropylene, polyglycolide, polylactide, polydioxanone, steel
Monofilament	*Multifilament*
Polyamide, polypropylene, polyethylene, polydioxanone, Catgut, steel	Polyester, polyamide, polyglycolide, polylaccide, silk, cotton, linen, steel
Braided	*Twisted*
Polyester, polyamide, polyglycolide, polylactide, silk	Cotton, linen
Coated	*Uncoated*
Polyester, polyglycolide, polylactide, cotton, linen	Polyamide, polypropylene, polyethylene, Catgut, collagen, steel

Table 4

Ph Eur Vol III/BP 1973 Gauge metric	Ph Eur Vol III/BP 1973 Diameter limits mm	Ph Eur Vol III/BP 1973 Knot pull kg	USP XIX Gauges	USP XIX Gauges	USP XIX Diameter limits mm	USP XIX Knot pull kg
0.1	.010–.019	—	—	0.1	.010–.019	—
0.2	.020–.029	—	—	0.2	.020–.029	—
0.3	.030–.039	0.010	9/0	0.3	.030–.039	0.023
0.4	.040–.049	0.025	—	0.4	.040–.049	0.034
0.5	.050–.069	0.040	8/0	0.5	.050–.069	0.045
0.7	.070–.099	0.070	7/0	0.7	.070–.099	0.07
1	.100–.149	0.150	6/0	1	.100–.149	0.18
1.5	.150–.199	0.350	5/0	1.5	.150–.199	0.38
2	.200–.249	0.650	4/0	2	.200–.249	0.77
3	.300–.349	1.25	3/0	3	.300–.339	1.25
3.5	.350–.399	1.60	2/0	3.5	.350–.399	2.00
4	.400–.499	2.25	1/0	4	.400–.499	2.77
5	.500–.599	3.00	1	5	.500–.599	3.80
6	.600–.699	3.75	2	6	.600–.699	4.51
7	.700–.799	4.75	3	7	.700–.799	5.90
8	.800–.899	6.25	4	8	.800–.899	7.00

many cases as much as 30–40% lower than the former. In practice, however, when a suture is placed in the tissues, the effective tensile strength of a suture is twice the tensile strength of the material used, since two sides of a loop are formed and both sides are contributing to the effective strength. Figure 6.2 shows in general terms the strongest, the weakest and the intermediate strengths of suture materials.

Tissue reaction

Tissue reaction to a material occurs for three reasons (Figs 6.3; 6.4; 6.5):

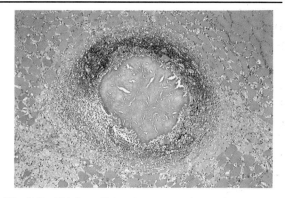

Fig 6.3 Brisk, cellular tissue reaction to Catgut at 3 days.

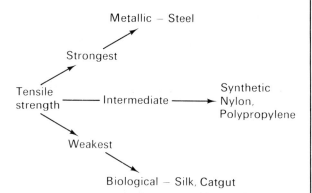

Fig 6.2 Relative strengths of suture materials.

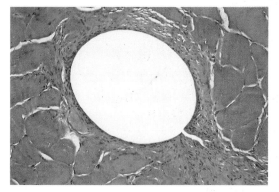

Fig 6.4 Bland tissue reaction to polypropylene at 28 days with minimal cellular reaction.

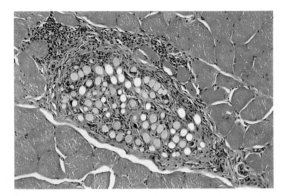

Fig 6.5 Tissue reaction to a braided synthetic absorbable material at 49 days. There is invasion of the braid by macrophages and giant cells.

1 The reaction to the trauma of implantation of the material and this occurs within 0 – 3 days.
2 The reaction to the material dependent partly on its physical shape, i.e., whether it is monofilament or braided, and on the chemistry of the material.
3 There is the reaction of absorption. In general, the faster the absorption, the more brisk and cellular is the reaction.

Biological materials tend to stimulate a polymorphonuclear and macrophage type of reaction, while synthetics stimulate a macrophage and giant cell reaction. Figure 6.6 shows in general terms the greatest, least and intermediate reaction to materials.

A method which we have recently started using in our laboratory to get an early read-out of tissue reactivity is by using tissue culture

methods. When a material is applied against mouse fibroblasts, the area of cell death around the material can be accurately measured and hence gives an indication of toxicity or non toxicity of the material within 0 – 48 hours which, if this material had been implanted *in vivo*, would have caused a reaction which would have been confused with the tissue reaction to trauma (Fig 6.7). The area of cell necrosis can be accurately measured using a MOP or Manual Optical Processor.

Absorption

There are two mechanisms of absorption of suture materials. The first applies to Catgut and collagen where the absorption mechanism is by enzymatic digestion. A proteolytic enzyme is carried in the lysozomes of the polymorphonuclear cell and these are released to attack the Catgut or collagen. The other mechanism is one of hydrolysis, which is the effect of water on the suture material and does not require the same cellular involvement as does Catgut with its proteolytic digestive enzymes. Hydrolysis is simply the action of water on a material causing breakdown. Hydrolysis is increased with rise in temperature or with pH changes. Figure 6.8 shows in general terms the comparative absorption times for Catgut, Dexon® (homopolymer of glycolide), Vicryl® (copolymer of glycolide and lactide) and PDS® (polydioxanone). As the material absorbs it loses tensile strength.

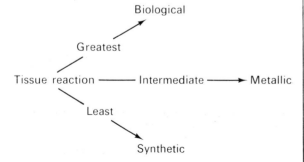

Fig 6.6 Graded reaction to suture materials.

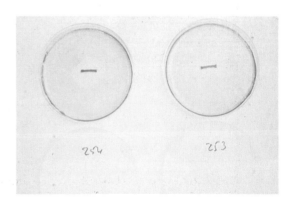

Fig 6.7 Comparison of two suture materials. In (a) there is a high degree of cell death and in (b) there is minimal cell death.

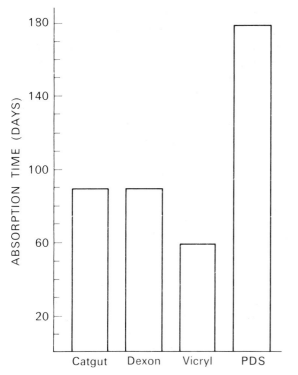

Fig 6.8 Comparative absorption times for Catgut, Dexon, Vicryl and PDS.

Figure 6.9 shows the comparative loss in tensile strength of Catgut, Dexon, Vicryl and PDS.

Knotting properties

There are several aspects of knotting of suture materials to be considered. First the ease with which a knot can be tied and this is dependent on the slipperiness or smoothness of the surface which is measured as the coefficient of friction. Next, there is the consideration of the material remaining securely knotted after the knot has been formed and this again depends upon the coefficient of friction of the material. The smoother the material the lower the coefficient of friction and, therefore, the easier it will be to slide through tissues and also to form a knot. Unfortunately, the smoother it is, the more readily it will become undone by slipping. The higher the coefficient of friction, the more difficult it is to pull the material through the tissues, but its knot holding capacity is very much greater because the rough surfaces prevent slippage. Another consideration in knotting is the memory or the spring-back of materials and, therefore, it is important when tying a surgical

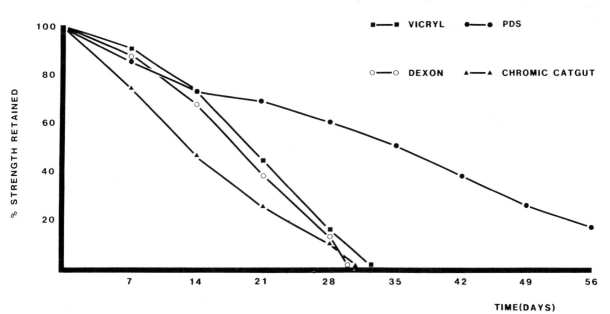

Fig 6.9 Comparative loss in tensile strength of Catgut, Dexon, Vicryl and PDS.

knot to make sure that spring-back and memory are overcome. The first throw when forming a knot should be a double throw and should be tied with sufficient tension to perform the task for which this suture or ligature is required, that is to stop bleeding or to appose cut surfaces. Care should be taken that when this tension is removed from the first throw that the suture does not spring back and thereby slacken off. The second throw is to lock the tension of the first throw into position. Many surgeons on their second throw attempt to tighten the first throw by applying extra tension on the second throw. While this is possible with materials which have a low coefficient of friction, it is not possible with materials of high coefficient of friction and frequently postoperative haemorrhage is due to the surgeon not appreciating that he is not tightening his first throw by his second throw. Frequently, a third throw is placed for complete security, but beyond three throws the surgeon is merely creating a larger and larger foreign body which, as explained previously, could lead to extrusion of the material. Each suture material requires a particular tying technique. Various combinations of throws have been described for different types of suture materials. By putting on the wrong type of knot, the material can slip; frequently to the extent that the effective tensile strength of the knotted loop is only 10% of the original tensile strength of the material. One of the best knots for synthetic suture material, whether it is absorbable or non-absorbable, is the 'synthetic knot' which is a double throw followed by a single throw and completed by a double throw. Figure 6.10 shows in general terms knot stability of the best, worst and intermediate materials.

Handling properties

Although difficult to define accurately, this is frequently referred to by both suture manufacturers and surgeons as the 'hand' of the material. Basically, it means the comfort with which the surgeon feels the material in his hands and the ease with which he can use that material. Scientifically, it can be measured by the use of Young's modulus or extension to break, but it is basically a feeling of security with the material while in use. Figure 6.11 shows, in general terms, the best, worst and intermediate handling properties.

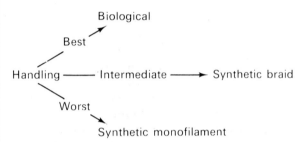

Fig 6.11 Relative handling properties of different suture materials.

Sterilisation

Modern surgical materials are presented to the surgeon already prepacked and sterilised. Basically, there are two methods of sterilisation, one by the use of 2.5 Mrad gamma irradiation from a cobalt 60 source, and the other method is by the use of ethylene oxide gas. The choice of which method is used to sterilise any particular material is dependent on the chemistry of the material. Basically, the more modern synthetic materials are sterilised by ethylene oxide since gamma irradiation tends to depolymerise these materials.

Catgut

Catgut is the oldest suture material known to man. It is made from the submucosa of sheep intestines or from the serosa of beef cattle intestines. The excised intestine is mechanically

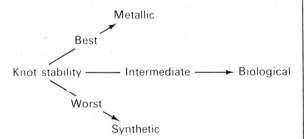

Fig 6.10 Relative knot stability of different suture materials.

cleaned to leave only the submucosa which is then known as the casing. The casings are split longitudinally to produce ribbons which are twisted together slowly under tension to produce a suture material. There are two kinds of Catgut — chromic Catgut, which has been treated with a chrome solution prior to twisting, and plain Catgut which is not chromicised. The function of the chrome is to tan the material and delay absorption. Chromic Catgut takes approximately 70 – 100 days to absorb, while plain Catgut absorbs in approximately 50 – 60 days. The fact that there is material in the tissues does not mean that material has tensile strength, since absorption rate and tensile strength loss are not synonymous. Chromic Catgut retains its tensile strength for approximately 30 – 32 days, while plain Catgut has lost all its tensile strength by approximately 20 days. Allergenic reactions to Catgut occur very rarely and many of the papers published in the past probably refer to iodine sensitivity, when the gut was sterilised with iodine. Catgut today is sterilised by either gamma irradiation or ethylene oxide. Tissue reaction differs between plain and chromic Catgut. Plain Catgut elicits an early lymphocytic intense reaction within 24 hours of implantation, while chromic Catgut produces a much slower polymorphonuclear reaction taking up to 3 days to become fully established. Catgut is easy to handle and knots well. In the chromic form the suture can be used safely in potentially infected cases, since the material will absorb rather than form a sinus and be extruded.

Collagen sutures

These sutures are made by extruding homogenised Achilles tendon of beef cattle which is almost 100% pure collagen. This material behaves in the same way as does Catgut and is made in plain and chromic form. In the larger sizes, however, handling is more difficult as the material is stiffer than Catgut.

Synthetic absorbable suture materials

One of the biggest breakthroughs in suture technology over the past 10 years has been the introduction of the synthetic absorbable sutures. These man-made fibres have a much less brisk tissue reaction than absorbables of biological origin and have a much more predictable tensile strength loss. At the time of writing there are three available synthetic absorbable sutures, namely Dexon (homopolymer of glycolide), Vicryl (copolymer of glycolide and lactide), and PDS (homopolymer of polydioxanone). Each of these materials will be described in turn.

Dexon

Dexon is the homopolymer of glycolide and is made by polymerising glycolide to form a long chain polymer. It is braided and is presented as a beige or as a green coloured material. It is coated with an absorbable material which allows easy emplacement of the suture. It absorbs in approximately 60 – 90 days and has lost all its tensile strength in approximately 30 days. It is sterilised by ethylene oxide.

Vicryl

Vicryl is a copolymer of glycolide and lactide in the proportions of 90% glycolide and 10% lactide. It is a long chain polymer in which the lactide elements intersperse randomly with the glycolide elements. It is presented as a beige or as a violet coloured material and is either uncoated or coated with a mixture of glycolide and lactide and calcium stearate. The addition of the coating allows it to slide through the tissues more readily and to knot more easily. It absorbs in 60 – 90 days and retains its tensile strength for approximately 30 – 32 days.

In the uncoated form, when using Dexon and Vicryl, it is important to ensure that tension is correct on the first throw of the knot since the second throw will not allow tightening of the first. It is sterilised by ethylene oxide.

PDS

PDS is the homopolymer of polydioxanone. Again it is a long chain polymer and, like Vicryl and Dexon, is made up of carbon, hydrogen and oxygen. This material is produced in the monofilament form, has a low coefficient of friction and, therefore, slides through tissues readily, but has knot security because the surface of the material, like polypropylene, tends to deform on knotting and hence maintain knot security. It absorbs in approximately 160 – 180 days and has lost all its tensile strength in approximately 56 – 60 days. It is sterilised by ethylene oxide.

All synthetic absorbable sutures break down by hydrolysis, as explained earlier and the end products of this degradation are carbon dioxide and water. Carbon dioxide is excreted in the expired air and the accompanying water is excreted both in the expired air and in the urine.

Natural non-absorbable suture materials

Silk

Silk is derived from the cocoon of the silkworm larvae. It is basically a protein like the keratin of hair and skin and is covered initially by an albuminous layer. This albuminous layer is removed by a process of degumming prior to making sutures. The suture is braided round a core and coated with wax to reduce capillary action. The material has high tensile strength which is probably totally lost after 2 years. Tissue reaction is greater to silk than to the synthetic non-absorbables because silk is a foreign protein. The cellular reaction is usually polymorphonuclear and is less intense than catgut. Encapsulation of the silk with a fibrous capsule usually occurs in 14 – 21 days. Handling properties are probably best of all suture materials and it knots easily and securely. It is sterilised by gamma irradiation.

Linen

Linen is made from flax fibres and is a cellulose material. It is twisted to form a fibre to make a suture. Tissue reaction is similar to silk and the material handles and knots well. It gains 10% in tensile strength when wet and is fairly unique in this respect. It is sterilised by ethylene oxide.

Cotton

Cotton is derived from the hairs of the seed of the cotton plant. Like linen, it is twisted to form a suture. The tissue reaction is like silk and linen and tends to be polymorphonuclear in type. Handling is good, but not as good as silk. It is sterilised by ethylene oxide.

Synthetic non-absorbable suture materials

Polyesters

Polyesters are probably better known as terylene and dacron. They are chemically extruded from a polymer and braided to form sutures. They have extremely high tensile strength and relatively low tissue reactivity. Tensile strength tends to be retained indefinitely. Passage through tissue is easy and is facilitated by the addition of a coating of polybutylate. However, because of the low coefficient of friction which gives it an easy passage through tissues, knot security requires that a third throw on the knot is advisable to prevent subsequent knot slip. Sterilisation is by gamma irradiation.

Polyamides

These are better known as nylon. They are chemically extruded, but this time generally in a monofilament form. Passage through tissue is easy because of low coefficient of friction and tissue reaction is minimal. Tensile strength loss after 2 years implantation is approximately 25%. The fibre tends to be stiff for handling, although this has recently been improved by the addition of fluid to the suture in the packet. Nylon also has a memory and hence knot security is lower than terylene. However, by placing three or four throws in the knot, security is assured. The future may well bring ultrasonic welding of the nylon suture to secure the knot and hence prevent slip. Sterilisation is by gamma irradiation.

Polyolefins

This fibre is better known as polypropylene. It is a monofilament and is chemically extruded from a purified and dyed polymer. It has an extremely high tensile strength which it retains indefinitely on implantation and an extremely low tissue reactivity. It can extend up to 30% before breaking and hence is useful in situations where postoperatively some 'give' is required on the part of the suture to accommodate for postoperative swelling. Handling is good and knotting very secure, since the material deforms on knotting and allows the knot to bed down on itself. It has a low coefficient of friction and slides through the tissue readily. It is sterilised by ethylene oxide.

Steel

In the monofilament form this material has high tensile strength and low tissue reactivity. Knot security is good and it pulls through the tissues easily. Handling, however, is difficult and it fractures readily when kinked. It is sterilised by gamma irradiation.

As already stated, surgical technique is far more important than the suture material used. However, a better understanding of the properties of suture material coupled with an understanding of wound healing can lead the surgeon to a more scientific approach to suture selection and more uniform surgical results.

Chapter 7

Which Dressing and Why?

T. D. Turner

PURPOSE AND FUNCTION

Throughout history, wounds have been dressed to assist in their healing. A great variety of preparations and products have been used, ranging from the hot oils and waxes of the early Egyptians to the animal membranes and faeces of the Middle Ages. The Linteum of the 1650s and the cotton and gauze tissue invented by Sampson Gamgee 100 years ago are still used today (Fig 7.1).

Until the 1960s there had been a minimum of research and development into wound man-

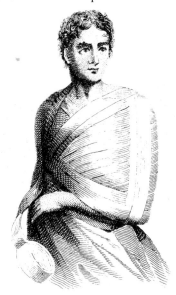

Fig 7.1 Wound dressings in 1859.

agement products and the materials available would have been easily recognisable to a surgeon of the late nineteenth century. Only in the last decade has consideration been given to the purpose and function of wound dressing procedures and, subsequently, products have been manufactured to fulfil these functions and have improved the speed and effectiveness of wound management.

The variety of available dressings is now greater than at any other time and is increasing each year. The standard 'dressing pack' which assumed a 'standard' wound can no longer embrace the range of products which have been designed for specific wound management problems. We are now reaching the point where it will be possible to 'diagnose' the wound and 'prescribe' the dressing and associated procedure.

The normal mechanism of wound healing has already been described. The four stages of repair were identified as inflammatory phase, destructive or cleansing phase, proliferation phase and the phase of maturation. These stages occur in both incised and excised wounds, the incised wounds healing by first intention and the excised, with their associated tissue loss, resulting in an extended healing process and maturation phase.

The biochemical and cellular activity leading to repair will proceed at a rate related to two principal factors; first, the general physiological state of the patient and second, the specific nature of the microenvironment of the wound. The optimum 'wound climate' would allow maximum activity of enzymatic and cellular systems.

The migration of activated fibroblasts and macrophages, the production of granulation tissue, the proliferation of endothelial cells and the completion of epithelisation will all contribute to the healing process. The management of the wound should neither retard nor inhibit any part of this process. The procedure used and the dressing applied must, therefore, contribute to the production and maintenance of an environment as close to the optimum as possible.

The problem of obtaining and maintaining the optimum environment will vary according to the nature of the wound. For example, the surgical incision will be easier to manage than the surgical excision. Again, a burn will be markedly different from a decubitus or ischaemic ulcer. There are, however, certain 'general' performance parameters which a 'general' dressing must possess if the optimum microenvironment is to be produced (Table 1).

Table 1
THE OPTIMUM DRESSING

1 To maintain a high humidity between the wound and the dressing
2 To remove excess exudate and toxic compounds
3 To allow gaseous exchange
4 To provide thermal insulation to the wound surface
5 To be impermeable to bacteria
6 To be free from particles and toxic wound contaminants
7 To allow removal without causing trauma during dressing change

Humidity levels and removal of exudate

The maintenance of a high humidity between the wound and the dressing contributes to rapid epidermal healing. A drying wound will result in a gas impermeable scab and will require epithelial penetration to a moist lower level (Fig 7.2). This will give extended healing times. Removal of excess fluid in the form of exudate avoids tissue sloughing. Exotoxins or

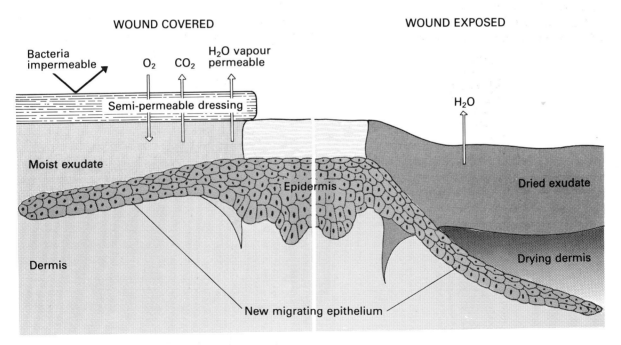

Fig 7.2 Difference between covered and exposed wound.

cell debris which may retard growth or extend the inflammatory phase will be removed along with the excess exudate. The balance between humidity and absorption is critical. Excessive wicking must be avoided to prevent drying and an optimum hydrophilic/hydrophobic absorption gradient is required.

Gaseous exchange

Gaseous permeability will allow water vapour transmission which is particularly important where there is a high body-fluid loss as in burns. Of equal significance to all wounds will be the effect of gaseous exchange on oxygen (Po_2) and hydrogen ion (pH) levels; movement across the dressing of oxygen and carbon dioxide will directly relate to the movement and activity of the cellular and humural factors previously mentioned. Epithelisation of the wound, in particular, is greatly accelerated by the availability of oxygen. The oxygen dissolves in the serous exudate and can be directly utilised by the migrating epidermal cells.

Thermal insulation

Thermal insulation will assist in maintaining the wound temperature at a level as close to body core temperature as possible. Phagocytic and mitotic activity are particularly susceptible to temperatures below 28°C. Thermal insulation and 'warm' dressing change conditions are very important if the optimum healing rate is to be maintained. Long exposure of wet wounds during dressing changes may reduce the surface temperature to as low as 12°C. The recovery of the tissue to full mitotic activity can then take up to 3 hours. Temperatures of 30°C and above may be found beneath a good insulating dressing and this will result in high mitotic activity with rapid epithelisation and improved granulation.

Impermeability to micro-organisms

Bacterial impermeability has a dual role. The wound will not heal if it is heavily infected. The inflammatory phase will be extended and, unless topical or systemic antibacterial agents are used, a more general infection will result. However, a limited number of micro-organisms are tolerated by most wounds and the destructive or cleansing phase will result in a self-sterilised environment produced by the activity of the phagocytes. The wound should now be protected from secondary infection and, if still contaminated, be prevented from transmitting the infecting organisms.

A dressing should, therefore, be impermeable to airborne micro-organisms which may fall on its surface and penetrate to and infect the wound. It should also act as a barrier to any wound organisms which may be transferred to the dressing surface and become airborne and thus cause cross-infection. This organism transmission occurs most frequently in dressings which exhibit 'strike-through' of exudate to the surface, providing a wet pathway to or from the wound surface. The passage of organisms can take as little as 6 hours from the time of strike-through; thus a barrier in terms of a water impermeable film, associated with the dressings, will reduce the possibility of strike-through occurring.

Freedom from particle and toxic wound contaminants

Both particles and toxic compounds which may contaminate a wound will be responsible for disrupting the healing pattern and possibly producing abnormal scar tissue. The incorporation of fibrous particles into a wound may result in a granuloma which could subsequently reduce the wound strength and induce keloid scarring. Particulate contamination can also reduce the infection resistance levels by a factor of 10^{-6}, thus organism levels which would previously have been self-sterilisable are infective and colonise the wound to produce a gross infection.

Trauma during dressing change

The wound environment may be optimally maintained with a product which has the preferred performance parameters but, nevertheless, is disrupted during the dressing change. The hazards of temperature change and secondary infection may be accompanied by a secondary trauma caused by the dressings adhering to the wound and, on removal, stripping newly formed tissue.

This adhesion is normally caused by the nature of the drying exudate and the trauma can be exaggerated on removal by the destruction of capillary loops which have penetrated the dressing material. This produces a bleeding surface which, at most, may revert the wound to the primary inflammatory phase and at least delay epithelisation.

Optimum dressing

The optimum dressing should, therefore, be a sterile, non-toxic, air-permeable product with a non-adherent surface, a predetermined absorptive capacity and hydrophilic/hydrophobic absorption gradient. It should be occluded by a water-vapour permeable, water and bacteria impermeable outer barrier. Although not associated with the micro-environment there are certain physical characteristics which the user will require to assist in the overall dressing procedure. The dressing should have:

1 A dimensional range to match the wounds.
2 An absorption range for dry and heavy exudate wounds.
3 Good conformability and good handle when both dry and wet.
4 Sterility and stability in storage and easy disposability.

Many of the early wound dressings were adapted from materials used for other purposes. Continued random development has produced dressings which, in general, meet only some of the requirements we have specified for a good healing environment. But frequently these dressings excel in a particular performance aspect. It is, therefore, difficult to identify a particular dressing as the only one suitable for a specific wound. In many cases it is the combination of knowledge, skill and experience of the staff concerned which results in the correct selection to produce the desired effect in the shortest time.

A knowledge of the products available and of the difference in their performance allows an informed selection to be made from among those dressings considered most suitable. We can, therefore, consider the available dressing products in a number of function-related groups.

PRELIMINARY TREATMENT

As already described, preliminary treatment of the wound may be necessary before the healing process can successfully progress; surgical debridement or mechanical cleansing may be required and systemic or topical antibacterial agents may be needed to control infection. A limited number of topical antibacterial medicated dressings are available.

These are generally leno cotton gauze products which have been impregnated with soft paraffin and antibacterial agents such as chlorhexidine, sodium fusidate or framycetin sulphate. They have the performance characteristics associated with simple paraffin tulle dressings. The paraffin prevents the dressing adhering to the wound and is particularly useful in controlling excess water loss in burns. It also partially insulates the surface against heat loss.

In addition to the burns application, the tulle gras dressing has been used as the wound contact layer in lacerations, abrasions, bites, puncture wounds and crush injuries. In ulcerative conditions such as varicose, diabetic, decubitus or topical ulcers, when used in the form of packing material, it has been reported to have promoted granulation. It is a good example of a product which excels in one parameter, namely non-adherence, but shows the absence of other performance criteria. This limitation has resulted in its replacement by other more specific products.

The incorporation of the non-systemic anti-bacterial compounds in the formulation will reduce wound infection and assist in the treatment of infected skin conditions such as eczema or dermatitis or prevent extensive infection in excoriated tissue around colostomies, ileostomies and tracheostomies. In use the leno gauze tulle dressing is the primary dressing or wound contact layer and is covered with an absorbent pad and retained in place with a tape or bandage. If non-adherence is the prime consideration then the oil-in-water impregnated viscose fabric product Adaptic® or the non-impregnated nylon fabric N–A® (Fig 7.3) may be used in place of the paraffin tulle dressing. N–A dressing in combination with povidone iodine is now available as Inadine® and provides an alternative to the traditional antibacterial tulles.

Many varied techniques are used to control

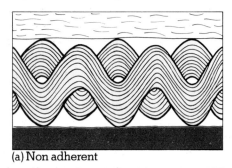

(a) Non adherent

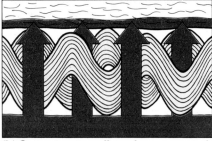

(b) Open structure allows free passage of exudate

Fig 7.3 N–A dressing. (a) non-adherent (b) open structure allowing free passage of exudate.

wound infection including irrigation chambers, impregnated ribbon gauze packing and topical applications but, with the exception of the above impregnated dressings, other antibacterial dressing products are designed to reduce infection by stimulating the wound defence mechanisms to produce a self-sterilising wound.

TYPES OF DRESSING

Early treatment methods included packing wound cavities with absorbent fibrous and woven materials including such products as gauze swabs, lint and the gauze and cotton tissue known as Gamgee®. More recently these have been joined by non-woven swabs made from viscose (rayon) fabric, for example Nu Gauze®. Both the gauze and non-woven swabs are available in 'filmated' form, that is where a layer of absorbent fibre is sandwiched between fabric layers to give greater absorbency.

These products are excellent absorbents, air permeable and good thermal insulators, but will overdry a wound. They are also no barrier to infection and will cause trauma on removal as a result of adherence and capillary loop insertion. However, the new non-woven fabrics show ever improving design/function characteristics which will result in more efficient products.

Undoubtedly, they do not promote wound healing, but they do retain their usefulness as cleansing pads and, in the case of ribbon gauze, as impregnated packing for heavily contaminated wounds.

Sleeve dressing pads

Sleeve dressing pads were designed to retain the absorption properties of the earlier materials and improve other aspects of performance. The simplest pads are constructed with an outer woven or non-woven fabric sleeve surrounding a cotton or viscose core. These pads are found in the standard 'Sterile dressing packs' and are a slight improvement over the fibrous absorbents and gauze and non-woven swabs. The wrap-around sleeve compresses the fibres and, therefore, produces faster absorption. It also results in a swifter strike-through giving a fluid pathway for the transmission of infective organisms.

Multi-layered pad

Multi-layered pads have been produced with more consideration of their function and with particular attention to adherence, absorption and strike-through; such products are Mesorb®, Surgipad® and Perfron®. They have fluid retardent layers in the upper part of the pad designed to delay strike-through. Additionally, in the case of Perfron, the layers of absorbent are interleaved with a tissue to improve the lateral dispersion of the serous exudate within the pad and this increases the total absorbent capacity of the dressing.

Although they do not possess moist interfaces and will lose particles to the wound surface, these dressings are an advance on the simple absorbents and can be used to advantage in heavily exuding wounds or as immediate postoperative dressings. They are available in a number of sizes and the larger sizes avoid the necessity of frequent dressing changes; or of using multiple small pads to cover one wound. The pads are kept in place by surgical tape or bandage.

In contrast to these high absorbency pads, there are low absorption capacity dressings which may be used for low exudate or drying wounds. These include products such as Melolin® and Telfa® which consist of thin fibre mixes sandwiched between two layers of perforated polymeric film, or one layer of film and one layer of non-woven fabric.

The polymeric film is placed in contact with the wound; its non-adherent character allows easy removal and the perforations allow for exudate transmission and aeration. Both pads show almost immediate strike-through and are therefore limited in their application by the degree and rate of exudate from the wound.

Island dressings

Melolin also appears as the absorbent pad located in the centre of an adhesive backing to produce the so-called 'island' adhesive dressing Airstrip®. The advantage of island dressings in use are that they completely cover the wound and avoid the necessity for bandages or tape to retain the dressing in position. Airstrip with its Melolin pad has an adhesive surround which is water vapour and air permeable. Band-Aid Fabric® and Steripad® have a butadiene foam pad with a non-adherent facing layer. The Steripad adhesive surround is perforated to allow the evaporation of excess fluid. These products are used primarily as immediate postoperative dressings.

Two-stage dressings

None of the dressings described so far fills all the requirements for optimum performance and, when the variety of wound types is considered, it is unlikely that all of the variables could be met satisfactorily by a single product. It is also unlikely that, in practice, all dressings will require all the performance parameters at each stage of the wound healing process or that certain of the parameters will be required other than in the first stages of the management procedure. For example, the osmotic gradient produced by Debrisan® may be an advantage in an infected cavity wound by producing the drying bio-environment unsuitable for the growth of micro-organisms. However, the same environment produced in a burn could well inhibit the development and migration of new epithelium. It is, therefore, logical to suggest that we may change the dressing type to match the step that we have reached in the wound healing procedure in the same way as we would modify a drug dosage regimen. Therefore, a dressing required in the first phase of healing may be replaced, to advantage, by a different product as the maturation phase is approached. The simplest way of taking advantage of the materials that are available is to adopt a two-stage dressing procedure where the wound contact layer, or primary dressing, could be designed and tailored to meet the specific parameters required for a particular wound.

An absorbent, air permeable, insulating pad may now be superimposed on the primary dressing to provide the second stage of the procedure. This latter pad can be selected to match both the rate and volume of serous loss. When saturated, the outer pad may be replaced without disturbing the wound contact layer. This will allow the healing process to continue with the minimum of interference.

In practice, the superpositioning of pads such as Surgipad on top of Melolin has recognised the need for such a system on exuding wounds. Products which can act as the primary dressing include Metalline®, Alutex®, Micropad® and Release®. Metalline and Alutex are slim absorbent pads faced with an aluminium metallised surface and described as non-adherent and claimed to improve the healing environment. They conform well, but do not possess the optimum permeability requirements. Micropad is a viscose fibrous laminate coated with polyethylene and is more efficient in maintaining a moist interface with the wound than other products of the same type.

Release is a newer product and is the first to

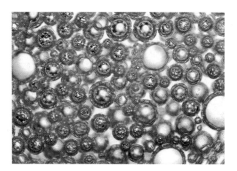

Fig 7.5 Photomicrograph of Synathaderm (x 100) showing closed cell structure.

identify wholly with the two-stage dressing procedure (Fig 7.4). It consists of a low density foam faced with non-adherent fabric and is recommended for use with a superimposed pad. The pad selected should be of the Surgipad type although with the optimum primary dressing even our displaced Gamgee might find a new application.

A more specific two-stage dressing is the recommended usage procedure associated with the product Synthaderm®. This is suggested for the management of full depth ulcer wounds associated with the lower extremities. This product is a closed cell, modified, foam sheet with a hydrophilic surface (Fig 7.5). The characteristics of the material closely approach the optimum primary dressing.

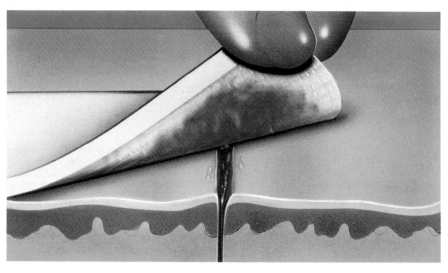

Fig 7.4 Non-adherent dressing — Release.

Semipermeable films

Dermabrasion and donor sites are characterised as shallow wounds which are known to produce intense pain. A dressing simulating the lost epithelium is most likely to be successful in producing rapid healing and reduction in pain. Such wounds can be treated optimally with homograft or heterograft materials such as lyophilised pig or bovine epithelium.

An alternative is to use a transparent, auto-adhesive, conformable polyurethane film which is permeable to water vapour and air impermeable to bacteria, particulate matter and water. Examples of such products are Op-Site®, Bioclusive® and Tegaderm®. Their conformability and permeability allow these types of dressing to be positioned over both large body areas and smaller angular areas. The wound response is similar to that found with Synthaderm, the moist surface encouraging rapid epithelisation of the debrided area with an immediate reduction in the pain levels. The extensible character of these films

and their tendency to produce a rapid increase in vascular supply make them useful products in the treatment of burns and in the prophylaxis and treatment of decubitus ulcers (Fig 7.6).

Polymeric materials

The foams were the precursors to a new family of polymeric materials such as Debrisan. This consists of straw coloured hydrophilic spherical beads 0.1–0.3mm in diameter which are composed of a dextranomer insoluble in water, but with an absorption capacity of four to five times its own weight (Fig 7.7). It will form a gelatinous layer in which the small molecules will be absorbed into the expanded bead matrix while larger molecules remain in the spaces between the beads.

The gel is formed with the wound exudate and an osmotic gradient results, reducing inflammation and associated oedema, absorbing micro-organisms and reducing bacterial contamination by initiating an osmotic gradient incompatible with the growth of bacteria. The

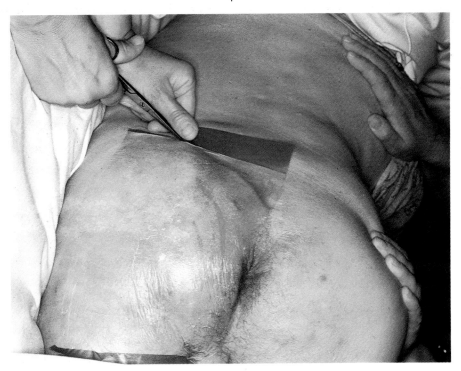

Fig 7.6   Op-Site used on a pressure sore.

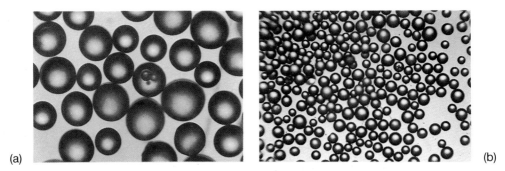

(a)   (b)

Fig 7.7 Photomicrograph of Debrisan (a) × 100; (b) × 37.

microenvironment for the production of gran-ulation tissue is improved and the result is a clean, debrided wound which is in the second phase of the healing process. The dressing is changed by removing the gel with sterile saline.

Debrisan may be used for small area burns, full depth wounds and indolent ulcers whether clean or infected. Its basic property is one of debridement, and once the granulation tissue is developing, its use should be discontinued in favour of one of the other environmental dress-ings. An important factor in the Debrisan treatment is its surface contact with all of the wound cavity. This has previously been diffi-cult to achieve without packing with a product such as ribbon gauze.

Debrisan is basically a polysaccharide and has been compared with the use of honey as a wound management product. An excised pilo-nidal sinus, anal fistula or wound dehiscence may lead to much larger cavities which are more difficult to manage and require extensive and intensive nursing.

A dressing has now been evolved for these wounds, in particular the production of a material called Silastic®. This is a silicon elastomer foam dressing. It is supplied as a fluid silicone base with a separately packed catalyst. When admixed, these form a low density, resilient elastomer and the mixture is poured directly into the wound, the resultant foam swelling to approximately four times the volume of the mixture.

This swelling will result in all parts of the cavity being brought into direct contact with the foam. The foam will absorb by accepting fluid into the surface cavities. When sufficient reduction of the wound cavity is obtained, the foam plug is discarded and a new dressing formed. This regimen can only be followed when the wound is free from gross infection.

Such a specific dressing emphasises the attention which is now being paid to the wound management area. New products con-tinue to appear: copolymer gels of radiation cross linked polyethylene oxide and water are now becoming available and are undergoing clinical assessment under the trade name of, for example, Vigilon®. Products described as second skin and synthetic skins are being recommended for particular applications. Af-ter the synthetic and semisynthetic polymers, the dressings of the future will almost certainly revert to biological type materials in combina-tion with synthetic products. Indeed, a pro-duct currently on trial consists of hydrophilic collagen peptides bonded to a silicone/nylon membrane.

It will eventually be possible to produce the optimum dressing for each type of wound and each phase of wound healing rather than rely on the all purpose 'out of sight out of mind' wound cover of the immediate past. The most advanced wound dressing consists of a pro-duct I have named 'Episyn': biodegradable, bacteriostatic, non-allergenic, tissue compati-ble synthetic skin, with the permeability and protective properties of homograft tissue. Un-fortunately at present nobody makes it.

TECHNOLOGICAL ASPECTS OF WOUND DRESSINGS

Peter Stevens

Dressings have changed greatly over past decades and now there seems to be a 'new improved' dressing appearing in the marketplace as frequently as the ever changing washing powders. Why has this happened? Technology has placed at our disposal many new materials, often with unusual or interesting properties. At the same time, our awareness of what is required to dress a wound, and precisely how a wound heals, is always improving.

Instead of our improved understanding of wound healing resulting in one dressing or device for all types of wound, the situation has arisen where each type of wound requires a special (optimum) environment. In short, we are coming into a whole family of dressings known as 'functionally specific dressings' each of which is recommended for a particular type of wound.

The problem, however, with functionally specific dressings is that they cannot, by definition, be used on all types of wound and, therefore, every new dressing requires a little more understanding in its proper use.

The result from the manufacturers' point of view is that a company wishing to develop more effective products must keep abreast of current technologies. In fact, unless they are able to evaluate new materials quickly, efficiently and accurately they would not be in a position to bring forward new products in an acceptable time to benefit the users (patients/nurses). For example, activated charcoal, which has been produced for many years in the form of powders and granules, became available as a woven cloth. The cloth was developed as a filter for the protection of personnel during chemical warfare and suggestions were made that it absorbed pollutants, including bacteria, out of water. Would this material adsorb the odours and bacteria associated with heavily infected discharging wounds?

A programme was set up to test the hypothesis in the laboratory. This was validated, product safety was established and clinical trials were arranged to prove the concept *in vivo*. Having proved the efficiency in use, the next phase was to develop optimal presentation to achieve maximum performance of the dressing in conjunction with pilot production and packaging trials. The evaluation of this unusual material was now complete and a new dressing (Actisorb Activated Charcoal Cloth®) was available for the treatment of heavily infected, discharging, malodorous wounds such as leg ulcers and fungating carcinomas (Fig 7.8).

Alongside the evaluation of new materials is the search for, and the development of, materials ideally suited to their intended use, whose theoretical characteristics are known, but are not currently commercially available.

Clinical evaluation is obviously an important part of development programmes, no matter how such previous laboratory work has been carried out. It is the first guide to the actual performance of the product in its intended use, and constitutes the basis of all further development work. From the trials, information is required as to the performance of the dressing, in terms of ease of application, absorbent properties, improved wound healing plus any special features of the particular dressing involved.

A look at the effect of these technologies on the development of dressings over the last few

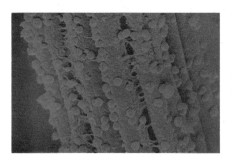

Fig 7.8 A photomicrograph of Actisorb.

decades shows an industry almost entirely textile-based, with products like lint, cotton wool balls, muslins and cotton gauze. Cotton gauze has, perhaps, been the least affected by the introduction of new technologies. From within the textile industry, however, a technology based around non-woven fabrics has developed and these materials are replacing gauze in many instances.

Perhaps a more marked change has taken place in the area of non-adherent dressings, where the first step of impregnating gauze with petroleum jelly has been followed by many products with different technology bases; for example — perforated polymer films, knitted continuous filament viscose rayon, polymer coated non-wovens, foams, heat treated thermoplastic fibres and metal foils or coatings. Finally, the development of adhesives to attach such products safely to the skin is yet another entirely separate technology.

Clearly, this is no more than a glimpse at some of the technologies involved in today's dressings. It would be true to say that as technologies develop and our understanding of wound healing continues to improve, so still more specialised dressings will appear in the future.

CLINICAL EVALUATION

Tim Coombs

Before any new wound dressing or wound healing device is introduced for general use, it must be tested exhaustively in laboratory and hospital environments. Clinical evaluation is the final and most crucial stage in the research and development process, and often represents the culmination of many years of effort on the part of research teams, clinicians and nurses.

Scientific approach

As dressings become more complex in design and function, so must the methods adopted for their clinical evaluation. There is a constant need for those conducting clinical trials to be both objective and impartial. This challenge is met in several hospitals through the establishment of specific units where clinical and nursing staff are trained in clinical research.

What, then, are the essential processes required to conduct a valid clinical trial? First, the objectives must be clearly defined and understood by all parties concerned. In the majority of studies they are the establishment of clinical safety and efficacy by a method consistent with the patients' best interests. They may be specific, such as a measurement of the absorbent capacity of a new dressing, or they may be more general, encompassing many attributes of dressing performance.

With the objectives firmly established and agreed, the next stage requires careful consideration since it involves the development of the detailed methods and the techniques to be employed to satisfy the objectives.

Within this framework, the techniques chosen must be scientifically rigorous and, wherever practical, precise measurements should be made rather than subjective statements of opinion. Effort expended at this stage will be more than rewarded by the value of the results obtained. A suitable control should always be employed, since this will provide a yardstick to which all test measurements may be related.

Hazards of bias

Bias can be a major problem in clinical trials if detailed thought is not devoted to its elimination in the design stages. If too much information regarding the performance expectations of the test product is relayed to those conducting the study, objectivity and impartiality are inevitably put at risk. The intelligent use of control will help minimise this problem and wherever possible 'blind' methodology should be employed.

In the simplest terms, 'single blind' studies do not reveal to the patient which is the test or control product and they cannot, therefore, choose between them on the basis of preconceived ideas and opinions. 'Double blind' studies take this process one stage further by concealing the identity of the test and control products from both patient and clinical investigator.

Bias may also be introduced by the way in which patients are selected for inclusion in clinical trials. The trial methods must show detailed inclusion and exclusion criteria by which patients are selected. It must also be stated how patients will be allocated at random to the test and control groups, or, if patients are to be asked to use both forms of treatment, the method of crossover to be adopted. There is always a minimum number of patients required to satisfy the method of analysis to be chosen and, therefore, it is always useful to have a statistician present at the design of the study.

A thorough statistical analysis of the results will be essential if the study is to achieve its main objective of convincing the medical profession of safety and efficacy. The analysis is applied so as to answer, with acceptable confidence, the question: 'Were the results obtained because of chance variations among the patients studied, or do they represent a real effect arising from the properties of the dressing or drug studied?'

Finally, the type and design of questionnaire or case report form used to record results is also part of the study methodology and should be easy and interesting to complete and, above all, unambiguous.

Road to success

When all aspects of design and methodology are agreed, the study protocol is drawn up to show precise details. This document is a central statement of the objectives, ethics and methods of the study and when signed by the manufacturers (or sponsors) and the clinical investigators becomes a contract of intent.

The successful initiation of a clinical trial is a most satisfying experience, not least because of its potential role in the alleviation of human suffering. Regular monitoring and recording of study progress are crucial to a successful outcome and everyone involved should study the protocol at the earliest opportunity.

Clinical investigators in the form of clinicians and nurses are key personnel in this process since they can provide 'first hand' knowledge and experience of the hospital situation, the patients' needs and the users' requirements.

Acknowledgement

Peter Stevens, PhD is a senior Project Scientist and Tim Coombs, PhD is Systems and Operations Manager with Johnson & Johnson.

Chapter 8

Wound Infection

Stephen Westaby and Sydney White

Despite an increasing number of preventative measures, infection and breakdown of surgical or traumatic wounds still accounts for a considerable amount of patient misery, prolonged hospital confinement and expense in nursing time, dressings and antibiotics. Wound infection remains as the commonest form of 'surgical' infection and surgery as we know it was only able to flourish after Lister's work on antiseptics.

DIAGNOSIS

Celsus' classic description of signs of infection in a wound still holds good today. The incision is inflamed, painful and tender to palpation and there is usually concomitant fever and leucocytosis. At times pus may exude around the sutures or from the incision or drain site. Fever, in the absence of other signs, should not immediately be attributed to infection at the wound site. Alternative causes of fever should be considered — drug reaction, pneumonia, urinary tract infection or infection at the sites of indwelling venous catheters. It must also be remembered that an element of redness and swelling is part of the normal wound healing process. Alternatively, infection in the deeper layers of a wound may cause fever before any local signs appear.

Clinical infection presents itself in various ways depending on the behavioural characteristics of different pathogens, the area of the body infected and pre-existsing local conditions (trauma, blood supply and so on). Systemic signs are not always specific and may vary with age. Although fever, tachycardia, leucocytosis and irrational behaviour are seen regularly in older children, the newborn seldom reveal such changes. Lethargy, refusal of feeds, jaundice and thrombocytopaenia may be the only indications of life threatening infections in the premature infant or full term newborn. Generally, if an infant fails to suckle or performs abnormally in any way after surgery, sepsis should be suspected immediately.

In the elderly or debilitated with impaired host responses, fever and local erythema may be absent and the first evidence of infection is generalised septicaemia (with subnormal temperature) or dehiscence of the wound which shows little or no attempt at healing (Fig 8.1).

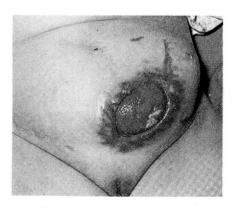

Fig 8.1 Wound dehiscence.

Infection may remain localised or spread to regional lymph nodes or distant areas. Direct extension is most common through subcutaneous tissue, fascial planes and muscle or tendon sheaths. Thrombosis of adjacent blood vessels may lead to necrosis, gangrenous changes and the likelihood of septicaemia. When bacteria are disseminated from an infected wound into the circulation, bacteraemia or septicaemia occur often leading to metastatic abscesses or secondary areas of infection. The incidence of septicaemia after wound infection cannot be stated as a single figure; it depends on the type and virulence of the organism, the extent of infection and the condition of the patient.

PHYSIOLOGICAL EFFECTS

Severe general physiological reactions may occur even while the infection remains localised. These include alterations in cardiac function, which may be depressed by toxins released by certain organisms such as clostridia, or elevated in the increased cardiac output which accompanies a rise in body temperature. There may be peripheral vasodilation with a fall in blood pressure and changes in the circulating blood volume. Renal function may be impaired and the lungs may suffer interstitial oedema and impairment of gas transfer (adult respiratory distress syndrome).

Many of these features result from activation of the complement cascade as part of the body's defence mechanism to the invading organism. Anaphylotoxins released in this process are beneficial when contained in a local inflammatory reaction, where they cause increased capillary permeability and attract white cells. When released in large quantities into the general circulation, they are extremely dangerous.

A prolonged febrile illness results in anorexia, decreased nutrient intake and increased catabolism, a combination of factors which results in rapid weight loss, decreased resistance to the infective process and poor wound healing. The temperature regulating mechanisms cause heat loss by sweating which, in turn, produces dehydration. It is, therefore, important to maintain calorie and water intake in patients with wound infection.

INCIDENCE

The incidence of wound infection after surgery ranges from 1% for 'clean' operations (after elective surgery not involving the gastrointestinal or urinary tract) to 40% after frank bacteriological contamination of the operative field by faeces or pus.

Clinical definitions of the degree of contamination are listed below and an analysis of the infection rates for each type in a large general hospital are shown in Table 1. Bacteria, of course, are the basic cause of wound infection, but they represent only part of the aetiology. In fact, every operation becomes contaminated to some degree by airborne or other micro-organisms, but relatively few become frankly infected.

Table 1
ANALYSIS OF INFECTION RATES RELATED TO WOUND TYPES

	Number of patients	Number of infections	%
Clean	47054	732	1.5
Clean-contaminated	9370	720	7.7
Contaminated	4424	676	15.2
Dirty	2093	832	40.0

Types of wound

Clean wound
Non traumatic, uninfected operative wound in which neither the respiratory, alimentary or genitourinary tracts or the oropharyngeal cavity are entered. Clean wounds are made under aseptic conditions and may be closed primarily without drains.

Clean-contaminated wound
Operative wound in which the respiratory,

alimentary or genitourinary tract is entered without unusual contamination.

Contaminated wound

Fresh traumatic wounds, operations with a major break in sterile technique (such as open chest cardiac massage) and incisions encountering acute non-purulent inflammation such as cholecystitis, cystitis or inflamed skin. Wounds opening the colon belong in this category.

Dirty and infected wounds

These include old traumatic wounds and those with clinical infection of perforated viscera. The organisms causing postoperative infection are already present in the operative field before operation.

SOURCE

Sources of infection are either endogenous or exogenous. An endogenous source is one in which the patient's own commenals (or normal bacterial flora) invade the wound and cause infection. These surface organisms are normally non-pathogenic, but can become pathogenic if they are permitted to contaminate the patient's wound. Endogenous infections often arise through the carelessness of nursing and medical staff in preparation of the patient for surgery or during dressing changes. Wound infections following surgery on the bowel can occur if the bowel contents are spilt into the peritoneum and wound at the time of operation. Patients may also contaminate their own wounds through poor personal hygiene.

An exogenous infection is one in which the offending organism is acquired from a source outside the patient's body. The organisms responsible for these infections may be carried either directly or indirectly into the wound. This transfer, which is referred to as cross-infection, may be caused by staff and other patients and also by surgical instruments. An example where direct transfer of micro-organisms into a wound can occur is when the

sterile surgical gloves of a staphylococcal carrier (surgeon or nurse) become punctured and the offending micro-organisms are shed directly into the wound. Indirect transfer of micro-organisms occurs through an intermediary such as contaminated surgical instruments and, to a lesser extent, through the environment in the operating room.

Cross-infection may also occur in the ward dressing-room when contaminated hands and instruments transfer micro-organisms from one patient to another during dressing changes. Airborne micro-organisms can also be carried from patient to patient and contamination can occur if no interval is allowed between different wound dressing changes.

Common micro-organisms

The human body is a reservoir of potentially pathogenic organisms. It is also an excellent host for invasive organisms providing not only nutrients but also protection from the harsh external environment. While many micro-organisms are quite capable of surviving hostile conditions by developing into spores or encapsulating themselves, they find the human body an ideal environment in which to flourish. They may then be responsible not only for wound infections, but for a great many other conditions such as respiratory, intestinal and urinary infections.

Aerobic bacteria proliferate in the presence of oxygen though many are able to grow in its absence. *Staphylococcus aureus* is present in the nose of 20–30% of normal persons and is re-

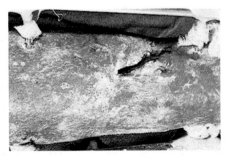

Fig 8.2 *Staphylococcus aureus* wound caused by compound fracture of tibia and fibula.

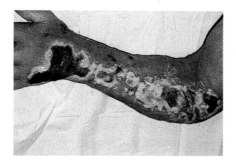

Fig 8.3 *Beta haemolytic streptococcus* Group A wound caused by a thorn prick on back of hand during gardening.

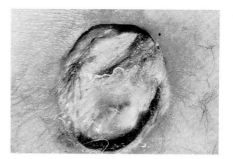

Fig 8.4

sponsible for many hospital infections (Fig 8.2). *Staphylococcus epidermidis* is present on normal skin in large numbers.

Beta haemolytic streptococci (Lancefield group A) (Fig 8.3) are present in the throats of individuals suffering from tonsillitis. They are also present in approximately 5% of healthy people and can be responsible for outbreaks of puerperal sepsis in maternity units and may cause skin grafts to fail.

Esherichia coli and *proteus* normally live in the bowel of healthy individuals and may be responsible for wound infections occurring after spillage of the bowel contents during surgery. They may also colonise surface wounds such as bed sores (Fig 8.4).

Klebsiella and pseudomonas species may also be found in the bowel and may be responsible for infections following surgery on the genitourinary tract and respiratory tract in susceptible individuals. Both of these organisms are free living and can be found anywhere where there is moisture or stagnant water. They tend to multiply in lotions and antiseptics which have become contaminated.

Anaerobic bacteria live and multiply in the absence of oxygen and this enables them to live in the bowel or soil. *Bacteroides* are found in the bowel where they proliferate in great numbers without causing harm. However, they may be responsible for peritonitis and pelvic abscesses when the bowel contents leak into the peritoneal cavity. *Clostridium welchii* are spore-bearing bacilli found in the bowel and soil. They may cause gas gangrene in deep, dirty,

traumatic wounds or in the presence of foreign bodies such as orthopaedic prostheses, particularly if the blood supply at the site of operation is inadequate. Exogenous infection is rare, contamination usually occuring from the patient's own bowel flora.

Clostridium tetani spores are present in great numbers in the soil and, if traumatic wounds become contaminated, tetanus may develop.

FACTORS INFLUENCING THE APPEARANCE OF CLINICAL INFECTION

Clinical infection can be defined as the growth of an organism in a wound with associated tissue reaction and depends on the number of pathogenic organisms multiplied by their virulence and divided by the host's resistance. This is normally represented by the following formula:

$$\frac{number\ of\ organisms\ \times\ virulence}{host\ resistance}$$

The mere presence of virulent bacteria in a wound does not itself imply infection. Host resistance may be sufficient to quell the appearance of significant clinical infection. Colonisation is the growth of organisms in the wound, but without tissue response.

Routine cultures of clean, surgical wounds at the time of closure have been reported as positive in as many as 85% of cases. This means that nearly all wounds have some kind of bacteria in them by the end of the operation yet only a few become infected. Infection, therefore, represents an unfavourable balance between dose of organisms multiplied by virulence, but divided by host resistance.

Dose of organisms

Obviously, the greater the number of organisms implanted in a wound, the more likely the chance for successful invasion and infection. The risk of wound infection after appendicectomy increases in proportion to inflammation of the appendix (as we might expect if bacterial contamination is a major determinant of wound infection). Once the organisms are implanted into the wound the environment is perfect for bacterial growth. Infection can be minimised if wound management follows the undermentioned principles:

* Careful aseptic technique
* Removal of all debris, foreign bodies and dead tissue.
* Achievement of complete haemostasis.
* Gentle handling of tissues using the minimum of suture material.
* Obliteration of dead space during closure.
* Minimum operative time to avoid overlong exposure and consequent growth of the numbers of bacteria.
* Lavage of the wound with sterile saline or a mild antiseptic such as Betadine® before closure.

Note that, as yet, antibiotic prophylaxis has not been mentioned. Antibiotics must not be relied upon to compensate for surgical errors or carelessness in wound management and prophylactic antibiotics should be limited to the following types of operative procedure:

* For patients with valvular heart disease or cardiac valve prostheses to prevent bacterial endocarditis.
* In cardiac operations with heart-lung bypass.
* In orthopaedic procedures for fixation of compound fractures or implantation of foreign material such as total hip replacement.
* For vascular operations using prosthetic grafts such as fermoro-popliteal bypass.
* After penetrating chest, abdominal or head injuries.
* In emergency operations where there is an active infection elsewhere in the body.
* For gastrointestinal procedures where there is heavy local contamination as in gangrenous cholecystitis, perforated appendix or diverticular disease, or when a bowel anastomosis is performed on an unprepared bowel.
* Where surgery is performed on patients with altered host resistance as in anaemia, agammaglobulinaemia and chronic steroid or immunosuppressive therapy.

There appears to be no value in the use of prophylactic antibiotics in 'clean' surgical procedures. In contaminated operations they must be given within 3 hours of tissue contamination and preferably before the start of the operation. This will provide adequate tissue levels of antibiotic at the time when bacterial invasion occurs. Choice of antibiotic must take into account the nature of the expected offending organism. When the gastrointestinal tract is opened, antibiotics which suppress both aerobic coliforms and anaerobic bacteroides should be given. Though the oesophagus, stomach and small bowel are frequently regarded as clear of virulent organisms, this is not the case in the presence of malignant disease.

When the operating room environment or the patient's skin are the likely source of contaminants, as in most cardiac or orthopaedic operations, antibiotics active against aerobic streptococci and staphylococci should be employed. For colonic resection preoperative bowel preparation helps to reduce contamination and, again, mechanical cleansing is the single most important element, although no one would dispute the value of metronidazole and its role in prevention of wound infection in this type of surgery.

Virulence of infecting organisms

This reflects the organism's ability to invade and create infection despite the body's host defence mechanism. Gram-negative infections have definitely increased during the past 15 years and since the discovery and widespread use of penicillin and other antibiotics which control Gram-positive organisms, Gram-negative sepsis has become a serious threat to modern surgical practice. Prophylactic antibiotic therapy has also failed to prevent Gram-negative septicaemia particularly in poor risk patients.

Moreover, intensive or prolonged antibiotic therapy may currently be contributing to the origin and increasing incidence of Gram-negative sepsis in some cases with bacteria previously considered to have little or no virulence. Organisms particularly dangerous in wound infection are the haemolytic streptococcus and clostridium species, whose adverse effects result from production of powerful enzymes and toxins.

Host resistance to infection

The emphasis on prevention of postoperative or post-traumatic wound infection is too often centred on blind pretreatment with antibiotics instead of consideration of those factors, apart from bacteria, which directly influence host resistance and susceptibility.

These factors are both local and systemic. Local factors including haematoma, tissue damage by crushing or excessive cautery, and foreign bodies such as suture material, play an important role. One experiment in pigs showed that in devitalised muscle, fatal infection with *clostridium* was a million times more common in the presence of foreign material than in clean, devitalised tissue.

Impairment of blood supply by suture strangulation or damage to a major blood vessel can lead to cell death. Dead cells then become a nutrient culture medium which enhances the growth of organisms. They multiply freely since, in the absence of adequate vascularity, white cells cannot gain access in sufficient numbers to be effective. Such infections are often characterised by the presence of multiple bacterial strains participating in synergistic or symbiotic activities. Prophylactic antibiotics may suppress one organism allowing the others to proliferate unabated.

With increasing awareness of the limitations of prophylactic antibiotics the importance of local defence processes becomes more evident. The natural or acquired resistance of the wounded area depends partly on the type of tissue but particularly on its vascularity. Organisms which have been overcome in a previous infection are unlikely to invade the tissues again at this point, probably because of the action of regional lymph nodes with improved phagocytosis and intracellular killing of the organisms. Various tissues are known to have different powers of resistance — for example, the abdomen, thigh, calf and buttock are especially susceptible while the face, scalp and thorax tend to become affected less frequently.

However, resistance to infection in any area can be weakened by many systemic factors. One is age, with the lowest incidence of wound infection taking place when the patient is in his late teens or early 20s, a slightly higher incidence being noted in children; then progressively higher incidence with age exceeding the late 20s. This distribution may be related to the body's immune mechanisms. The various components of the body's host defence mechanisms interact in a co-ordinated way to control infection through a final common path, the acute inflammatory response. Defects of this response may be congenital, as in certain immune deficient states where antibodies are lacking, or acquired at the time of illness.

Failure to respond to an infective stimulus is known as anergy and recent research has shown that simple skin testing with recall antigens (materials which normally elicit an immune response) can be used to predict patients who are likely to suffer from postoperative sepsis and death. Anergy in surgical patients generally represents an acquired and reversible defect in host defences and successful management depends on early recognition of associated treatable states such as malnutrition, trauma, haemorrhage, shock and remote infection (places other than the operative site).

It has been well known for many years that certain nutritional and metabolic states such as chronic inflammatory bowel disease, diabetes, severe obesity, anaemia, dehydration or shock increase the likelihood of wound infection and deficiency of immune competence is the likely mechanism. Patients can be skin tested before operation and, if found to be anergic, can be investigated for various conditions which may be responsible.

Malnutrition is then corrected, if necessary, by total parenteral nutrition, systemic sepsis is treated appropriately and, if the patient remains anergic, postponement of elective major surgery should be considered.

PERIOPERATIVE FACTORS WHICH INFLUENCE THE INCIDENCE OF CLEAN WOUND INFECTION

As a rule postoperative wound infection has its origin during the surgical procedure, not as a result of postoperative cross-infection. The clean wound infection rate is the standard by which surgical technique and nursing preparation and aftercare must be judged. Overall infection rate is the figure commonly quoted in hospital statistics, but in many ways it has little meaning as it is closely related to the types of operation performed. If most of the operations in an institution are clean e.g. hernias or clean orthopaedic procedures, the overall infection rate will be low. If on the other hand, many operations are contaminated e.g. trauma and bowel operations, the incidence of infection will be much higher.

In general, a clean wound infection rate of less than 1% is exemplary, 1–2% is acceptable, but more than 2% is cause for concern. An acceptable level of clean wound infection can be achieved by a continuous effort to reduce contamination and adhere to the meticulous principles of wound care.

The analysis in Table 1 (p. 71) shows the overiding importance of endogenous contamination, for instance, where pus is encountered, infection is twenty times higher than in clean wounds. There is a steady increase in clean infection rate with increasing age, in patients with diabetes (10.5%), with obesity (13.5%) and with malnutrition (16.5%). This is largely the result of reduced host resistance which, in turn, reduces the dose of contamination required to produce clinical infection in these patients.

The following factors may be expected to influence the degree of contamination of clean surgical wounds:

Surgeon's hands
In 1847 Semmelweiss identified the hands of doctors and students as the vectors of infection in puerperal sepsis. He reduced mortality by insisting on hand washing with hypochlorite solution. These days surgical scrubbing with antiseptics is routine and in many hospitals in the USA this is timed strictly to 10 minutes.

Patient's skin
It has been shown that in the patient showered with hexachlorphane before surgery the clean wound infection rate was 1.3% as compared with 2.1% if he showered with soap and 2.6% without a shower. It is now routine to prepare the patient's skin with the preferred antiseptic solution preoperatively.

Shaving the operative site
It has been customary to shave the surgical site for many years, though recently critical examinations of this procedure has produced surprising results. In one survey the clean wound infection rate was 2.5% in shaved patients; in patients who were not shaved, but had the surrounding hair clipped, the infection rate was 1.7% and in those with neither, the rate was lowest at 0.9%. Another trial demonstrated an even greater difference of 5.6% for shaved patients and 0.6% for the unshaven. Superficial skin abrasions contaminated by endogenous staphylococci probably account for the infected

cases and recently there is evidence that male patients whose chests are shaved before cardiac surgery have a greater incidence of prosthetic valve endocarditis after valve replacement. Depilatory creams are a useful substitute when hair removal is required.

Plastic skin drapes

These have not reduced clean wound infection rates though they serve to fix the skin towels to surrounding skin without the need for metal clips.

Preoperative hospitalisation

The longer a patient stays in hospital before operation, the more likely he is to develop a wound infection. This probably results from skin colonisation by organisms to which he is not resistant. With a 1 day preoperative stay, the infection rate is 1.1%, with 1 week 2.00% and for more than 2 weeks 4.3%.

Diathermy

When electrocautery is used to cut subcutaneous tissue, the clean infection rate is double that for the scalpel. Additional diathermy coagulation close to the skin worsens the infection rate unless the bleeding vessel is carefully grasped by fine forceps. Excessive use of the diathermy leaves large amounts of dead tissue and burnt eschar in the wound which greatly adds to the risks of clinical infection. In contrast, haematoma formation is an even greater risk.

Wound drainage

This is employed to prevent haematoma formation, but may increase the rate of infection if used inappropriately (Table 2). The introduction of closed wound suction drains has been a significant advance.

Duration of operation

There is a direct relation between the length of operating time and the infection rate. The rate of infection for clean operations doubles with every hour. There are a number of explanations for this; firstly, the dose of bacterial contamina-

Table 2

Mode of drainage	Infection rate
No drain	2.2%
Penrose drain through stab wound	1.8%
Penrose drain through wound	8.8%
Closed wound suction drainage	0.6%

tion increases with time, wound cells are damaged by drying and retraction, and increased amounts of suture material and electrocoagulation reduce the resistance to infection. Also, longer procedures are more likely to be associated with blood loss and shock, thereby reducing the general resistance of the patient.

PATHOLOGICAL FACTORS INFLUENCING THE INCIDENCE OF WOUND INFECTION

Pathological factors which predispose to wound infection are as follows:

1 The type of wound and extent of trauma to tissues and organs during surgical intervention or injury. Some examples of this are contaminated wounds as in surgery on the gastrointestinal tract, gunshot wounds, or foreign material left in wound (i.e. gauze, suture materials, instruments, drains, or formation of a haematoma.) Other traumatic types of wound which are likely to become infected include compound fracture (Fig 8.2 pp. 72), burns, pressure sores (Fig 8.4, pp. 73), and leg ulcers.

2 Patients suffering from prolonged hypovolaemic shock resulting in hypoxia and subsequent cell death. Vascular insufficiency, from whatever cause, inevitably leads to infected lesions, especially in the lower limbs.

3 Poor inherent resistance to enable the patient to fight off infection. This may be due

to age, sex or chronic disease such as diabetes mellitus or leukaemia. Other less common diseases include bone marrow deficiency and scurvy (vitamin C deficiency).

4 Reduced resistance of the host by the administration of certain types of drugs will also lead to infections. These include immunosuppressants, steroids, cytotoxics and certain antibiotics.

5 Malnutrition and obesity also contribute to the likelihood of wound infection — malnutrition because of the lack of host resistance and the subsequent inability to fight infection, and obesity because of the poor vascular supply in tissues containing large quantities of fat cells.

6 Prolonged anaesthesia in major surgery especially that which involves the use of prosthetic devices. Among these are the deep seated wounds associated with replacement heart valves and new hip and knee joints. Organ transplantation also represents a particular hazard from an infection point of view. First the recipient is usually debilitated and, therefore, has a poor resistance to infection. The donor organ may unwittingly be infected at the time of transplantation and the use of immunosuppressant drugs prevents an appropriate host response.

PREVENTION

It is essential that early recognition and isolation of any source of infection is made and precautions are taken to prevent the spread of infection. Efforts should be made to remove the source of infection, or the patients from the source. Extra care is needed, when nursing patients with invasive devices such as central venous pressure lines, intravenous infusions or indwelling urinary drainage catheters, since such therapeutic devices provide a port of entry for harmful micro-organisms. Excreta and other body discharges must be disposed of safely and care must be taken to avoid contaminating wounds, the hands and the surrounding environment. When nursing patients with known infections, protective clothing should also be worn.

Aseptic techniques should be used for all wound dressings. This means sterile equipment and dressing materials together with a non-touch technique. Patients with known wound infections should have their dressings changed after those who have wounds which are clinically free of infection.

Used dressings and other ward refuse should be contained and disposed of in a safe manner by incineration. Soiled linen from infected patients should be bagged at the bedside and placed in the appropriately colour coded bags. An agreed colour code for methods of collection and disposal will make this procedure easier to follow (Fig 8.5).

Good housekeeping practices are essential in order to provide a safe and agreeable environment in which to nurse patients and to work. Thorough cleaning with a suitable detergent eliminates many potentially harmful micro-organisms by removing them. Cleaning equipment must be maintained in good working order so that it performs satisfactorily and does not cause the inadvertent spread of micro-organisms.

It should be remembered that every healthy person is capable of infecting himself and others and, therefore, good personal hygiene is essential. Personal hygiene is of major importance as it promotes health and limits the spread of disease, in particular those which are transmitted by physical contact. All personnel who are in direct and indirect contact with patients should make sure that they:

1 maintain a clean body by frequent washing with soap and water;

2 wash hands after using the toilet and prior to preparing or consuming food;

3 keep contaminated hands away from eyes, ears, nose, mouth and genitalia;

4 wash and dry hands thoroughly on individual disposable towels after handling patients;

Methods of disposal

Method		Destination
Bag (nylon)	Soiled linen	Laundry
Bag (alginate stitched) ⬤	Fouled/infected linen	Laundry
Bag ⬤	Refuse, including infected dressings, disposable nappies, I.V.I. giving sets (remove needles first)	Hospital incinerator
Bag ◯	Instruments and equipment for dressings for reprocessing	C.S.S.D.
Bag ⬤	Non-infected refuse, i.e. flowers, waste from offices, etc.	Disposal tip
Plastic container	Syringes, needles, ampoules, blades - all sharps	Hospital incinerator
Special bin	Aerosol cans, bottles and breakages	Disposal tip

Fig 8.5 Colour code for methods of collection and disposal.

5 avoid the common use of personal items such as toothbrushes and razors within the hospital.

To avoid the emergence of multiple-resistant strains of bacteria, it is necessary to discourage the empirical use and topical application of antibiotics. Prophylactic antibiotics, when indicated, should be given immediately before surgery and discontinued within 72 hours. Administration of antibiotics for the treatment of wound infections, where necessary, should be determined by microbiological tests which will isolate the infective micro-organisms and indicate which antibiotics may be effective. 'Blind' antibiotic therapy is rarely appropriate and may be counterproductive or frankly dangerous.

It should be remembered that antibiotics upset the normal bacterial balance of the body. This may cause an unpleasant and potentially dangerous overgrowth of organisms, such as *Candida albicans* (thrush), which is commonly found in the mouth and vagina. This is unpleasant for the affected patient and may lead to other patients becoming infected if adequate control measures are not taken.

The infection control team

The infection control team can make a valuable contribution to the prevention of wound infections. This can be in the form of advice, monitoring of patients and education of staff.

Advice concerning such topics as preoperative skin preparation, type and time of shave, skin antiseptics and hand degerming methods together with wound dressing techniques may be offered to all nursing staff.

Monitoring is practised by surveillance which means keeping a constant watch over every aspect of the onset and spread of infection. This practice demands observation of the patient, taking swabs for culture, methodical collection of relevant information, interpretation of the microbiological investigations and the identification of the causative bacterial strain. Monitoring is an essential method of infection control as it assesses the prevalence and incidence of infection. It also follows the course of an outbreak of infection and helps to trace the source. Therefore the inspection of all wounds should be carried out by the same person in order to gather accurate information and this is the province of the infection control nurse. The monitoring of personnel is undertaken to follow the course of an outbreak of infection and to help determine its source. This includes the screening of ward and theatre staff for the presence of skin and other infective lesions.

TREATMENT

The patient with a wound infection feels miserable because of the systemic effects described. His appetite is depressed by the unpleasant smell of the purulent discharge and the sight of his wound when the dressings are changed.

General nursing care, reassurance and encouragement are an important part of the management of any patient with wound infection. Adequate nutrition must be maintained despite loss of appetite, even if this requires nasogastric or parenteral feeding. Dehydration should be avoided in febrile patients and oral hygiene must be carefully maintained.

Local treatment of the infected wound

As a general rule the earlier the onset of wound sepsis the more destructive and life threatening the infection will become (Table 3). Treatment of the infected surgical incision is straight forward. The wound must be opened along the length of the infected part, the patient is then positioned so as to obtain reliably dependent drainage. If tissue necrosis is extensive, careful debridement should be performed.

Most infections are limited to the subcutaneous fat layers and fluctuation signals the appropriate time for drainage of most superficial abscesses. Once the wound is open it should be allowed to close spontaneously by contracture and granulation. Secondary suture is only rarely considered and resuture at the time of drainage is still strictly prohibited in postoperative infection, although some authors have advocated primary suture and obliteration of abscess cavities with antiobiotic cover.

Superficial wound abscesses may be lightly

Table 3
THE CLINICAL FEATURES AND BACTERIOLOGY OF WOUND INFECTION

Postoperative day of onset	Usual organism	Appearance of the wound	Systematic signs of infection
1–3 days	*Clostridium welchii* (gas gangrene)	Brawny oedema, cool haemorrhagic; intense local pain; may be gaseous crepitations; foul exudate	Sustained high fever (39°–40°); psychosis; delirium; occasional jaundice; leucocytosis: 15 000+
2–3 days	*Streptococus*	Erythema, warm, tender; serous exudate; sometimes haemorrhagic; cellulitis	High, spiking fever (39°–40°C); irrational at times; leucocytosis: 15 000+
3–5 days	*Staphylcoccus*	Purulent exudate or abscess; Erythema; warm, tender	High spiking fever (38°–40°C); irrational at times; leucocytosis: 12 000–20 000
5 days	Gram-negative rods	Purulent exudate; erythema; warm, tender	Sustained low graduating to moderate fever (38°–39°C); leucocytosis: 10 000–16 000
>5 days	Mixed 'symbiotic' organisms. Usually anaerobic plus Gram-negative rods	Erythema, warm, tender; purulent foul exudate; focal tissue necrosis	Moderate to high fever (38°–40°C); leucocytosis: 15 000+; Variable cerebral state.

packed with gauze after drainage, while deeper abscesses are kept open by rubber drains or sump tubes. The author favours continuous or intermittent topical irrigation with saline or mild antiseptic solutions instead of frequent, tedious dressing changes. Dressings rapidly become wet, soggy and offensive, macerate the skin and are unpleasant to replace for both nurse and patient (Fig. 8.6).

Skin care plays an important part in wound infection. Adhesive tape on excoriated skin causes further damage and should be avoided. Local moist heat relieves pain and increases blood and lymph flow. Heat may be applied by intermittent moist compresses which hasten localisation of pus. Prolonged heat should be avoided since it encourages oedema and satellite infection.

Appropriate parenteral antibiotics are required in addition to incision and drainage when there is evidence of septicaemia (systemic toxicity, high fever) or progression of infection despite adequate drainage. Systemic antibiotics are also indicated in conjunction with surgical drainage in all cases of intra-abdominal abscess. Antibiotics can be chosen initially on the basis of Gramstain and microscopy, before cultures have grown the responsible organism.

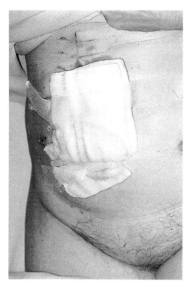

Fig 8.6 Wet, soggy and offensive wound dressing.

Purulent material (pus, debris, dead tissue) from the deepest aspect of the wound should be sent for aerobic and anaerobic culture and sensitivity studies. Generally speaking, *E. coli*, bacteroides and *B. fragilis* are the usual causes of wound sepsis following gastrointestinal or gynaecological surgery, while staphylococcus and pseudomonas predominate when intra-abdominal viscera have not been resected or opened.

Wound infection resolves rapidly when the wound has been opened and adequately drained. Irrigation usually expedites this and, when appropriately used, antibiotics contribute by preventing local spread and septicaemia. Allowing soggy dressings to sit in a purulent wound does little to encourage resolution of infection and, when removed, these dressings constitute a cross-infection risk.

SOME SPECIAL TYPES OF INFECTION

Necrotising fasciitis

A serious, spreading infection caused by haemolytic streptococci or staphylocci involving the fascial planes of wounds. It may be fulminating or lie dormant for a week or more before beginning its rapid spread, accompanied by tissue necrosis and resulting in gangrene. Treatment involves the excision of the entire area of fascial involvement, administration of large doses of penicillin and the appropriate systemic support.

Clostridial myonecrosis (gas gangrene)

An anaerobic infection of muscle causing profound toxaemia, extensive local oedema and necrosis and production of gas bubbles. The affected area swells and discharges foul, brown fluid. The muscles are first red and friable, progressing to a purple/black, pulpy mass. The overlying skin becomes blotchy and purple, then blackens and sloughs (Fig 8.7). Delay in diagnosis and treatment (often by amputation) is fatal; large doses of penicillin

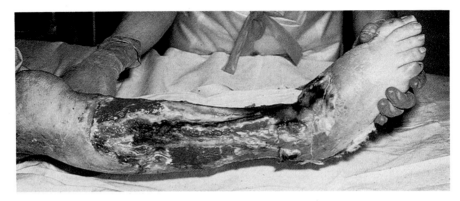

Fig 8.7 Gas gangrene.

are also given. Hyperbaric oxygen has been used to minimise spread of infection, but mortality ranges from 25–40%.

Bacterial synergistic gangrene (Meleney's gangrene)

A combination of non-haemolytic streptococci and aerobic haemolytic staphylococci which produce cellulitis followed by progressive gangrenous ulceration 7 to 14 days after infection. Treatment is by radical excision of the ulcerated area and large doses of penicillin.

Human bites

These are normally mismanaged in the accident department. Often contaminated by streptococci, staphyloccocci, bacillus and spirochetes, the original wound must be treated by debridement, cleansing and immobilisation. Systemic antibiotics, usually penicillin, must be used.

CONSEQUENCES

At the very least a hospital acquired wound infection complicates a patient's recovery, increases his discomfort and can prolong his stay in hospital often delaying his return to work. Wound infection may eradicate the desired effect of operations, for instance a herniorrhaphy may dehisce leading to recurrence, or laparotomy wounds result in incisional herniae (Fig 8.1). Skin grafts may fail to take and bowel anastomoses lead to fistula formation. Certain types of infection may lead to temporary or protracted disability, for instance in one case 15 infections occurred out of 25 eye operations performed in the same week and 6 patients lost the sight in one eye. Infection after vascular operations may necessitate amputation and run the risk of sudden exsanguinating haemorrhage. Septicaemia from postoperative wound sepsis may result in death, especially in the old and debilitated. Prosthetic valve endocarditis requiring re-replacement is a common consequence of wound sepsis after cardiac valve replacement.

The Public Health Laboratory Service Report (1960) showed that the consequence of wound sepsis in surgical patients was to increase the length of stay by 7.3 days. Five other studies in the previous 8 years made estimates of the increased length of stay from 2 to 60 days. A recent study on orthopaedic patients found that infections doubled the length of a patient's stay in hospital. Each prolonged stay means that another patient awaiting admission will have to wait longer. Subsequently patients take their resistant staphylococci out of hospital and may carry them for 6–12 months. Reinfection or cross-infection of other susceptible individuals may, therefore, occur at a later date.

Wound infection places an additional burden on the time and resources of the hospital

Table 4
ESTIMATE OF COST PER PATIENT OF HOSPITAL-ACQUIRED INFECTION

Type of hospital-acquired infection	Country	Year	Delay in discharge (extra days)	Cost per patient	Author
Surgical wounds	USA	1973	9.9 days (hospitalisation alone)	$600	Cruse & Ford
Surgical wounds	USA	1978	8–10 days	$15 000	Crow
Orthopaedic	Scandinavia	1963/7	Up to 54 days	2.5–5 times more than control patients	Lidgren
All infections in orthopaedic patients	United Kingdom	1978	Up to 17	£775	Davies & Cottingham

and its medical and nursing personnel. In addition one may have to resort to the widespread use of broad spectrum antibiotics which are expensive and have the disadvantage of risking the development of hospital resistant strains.

The combined expenses resulting from wound infection are very high. They include at least two components, first the additional hospital costs and second the additional loss of income to patients not insured against their extra stay in hospital. The figures in Table 4 show some recent attempts to estimate the costs per patient of surgical wound infection.

Chapter 9

Wound Sinus or Fistula?

William G. Everett

When there is a discharge of pus or other matter from any wound consideration needs to be given as to where this has arisen and why. A clear understanding of the cause of the discharge is fundamental to management and prognosis. Observation of the character and quantity of the discharge may suggest the site from which it has come. If this consists of a small amount of haematoma, it has probably come from a collection in the subcutaneous layers of the wound. Larger quantities of fluid clearly cannot collect in this limited space and must have come from a cavity deep to the wound, such as the abdominal or thoracic cavity, or the viscera contained in them. The discharge of serosanguineous fluid from a wound suggests disruption of the deeper layers and when the volume is large, and exceeds the amount which could possibly be contained in the subcutaneous layers, the diagnosis of wound disruption is certain. Sometimes the fluid will almost gush out when the patient moves or coughs and a defect in the abdominal wound can sometimes be palpated. The discharge of any unusual looking fluid from a wound — be it clear, bile-stained, yellow or brown — must raise the possibility of a fistula. A continuing discharge which does not arise from a fistula must be coming from a sinus.

A sinus is a track communicating with a deep-seated abscess. The deep end of the track is blind. Superficially the sinus opens into the skin (Fig 9.1). A fistula, on the other hand, is an abnormal track connecting one viscus to another or a viscus with the skin. The track, therefore, connects one epithelial surface with another.

WOUND SINUSES

Many wound sinuses are chronic and fail to

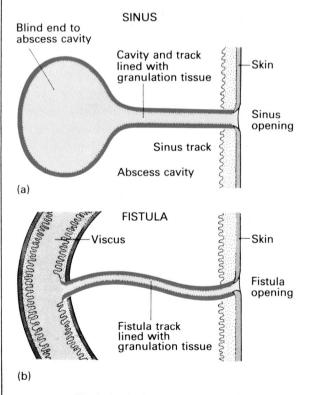

Fig 9.1 A sinus and a fistula.

heal because the abscess cavity contains some foreign material. Examples are the pilonidal sinus which contains hair and the sinuses of chronic osteomyelitis which fail to heal because of a sequestrum of dead bone. The commonest wound sinus is due to buried suture material. Sinuses are particularly likely to occur when braided non-absorbable materials are used to close contaminated wounds as the mesh of the material acts as a nidus for bacteria, where they can escape attack from macrophages. Infection and sinus formation can also occur around the knot of synthetic monofilamentous materials, particularly if the ends of the knot have been left long (Fig 9.2). As with all sinuses, the infection and discharge continues until the foreign body is removed. In the case of nylon, it is a simple matter in the Outpatient Clinic to pick up the knot with a crochet hook and cut it off. Healing quickly occurs and it is not necessary to remove all the nylon. Removal of braided material is more difficult and usually requires exploration under a general anaesthetic.

Dressings packed into an open wound may be retained and be a cause of that wound failing to heal. In treating sinuses, it is common practice to pack an open wound with ribbon gauze to prevent the wound edges from healing in too quickly, but this leaves a cavity which fails to drain adequately. Small lengths of ribbon gauze are not infrequently found in perineal sinuses, which persist after abdominoperineal excision of the rectum or proctocolectomy. Figure 9.3 illustrates the sinogram of a perineal wound which was left open following proctocolectomy and dressed with silicone foam elastomer (Silastic). The persistent sinus was due to part of the silastic 'bung' becoming detached (Fig 9.4). When this was removed the sinus rapidly healed.

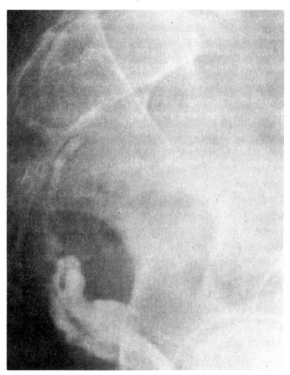

Fig 9.3 Sinogram of a perineal wound showing track leading up in front of the sacrum.

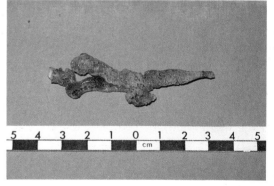

Fig 9.4 Piece of Silastic removed from the perineal wound.

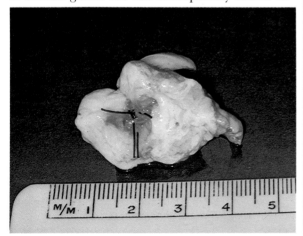

Fig 9.2 Stitch sinus occurring around a nylon knot.

Treatment of wound sinuses

A common cause of a persistent sinus is inadequate dependent drainage of an open wound — the cavity acting as a sump of chronically infected granulation tissue. Poor drainage usually occurs as a result of the skin edges healing too rapidly (Fig 9.5). The orifice of the sinus narrows down leaving a cavity which cannot drain satisfactorily and its contents, therefore, become infected causing a continuous or intermittent purulent discharge. This situation can be prevented by the surgeon making the opening of the wound sufficiently wide in the first place and by good nursing technique. The wound opening at skin level must be kept open by physically breaking down any adhesion that occurs between the edges. This can be done by packing the wound, but equally well by stretching the

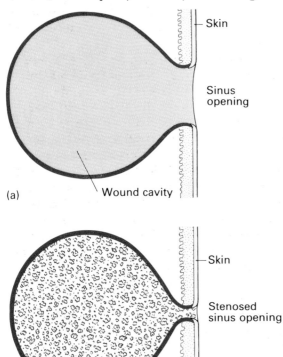

(a)

(b)

Fig 9.5 (a) A healing cavity; (b) Stenosis of the sinus opening causing retention of secretions and infection.

wound edges with a finger (covered by finger cot or glove). As has already been stated the disadvantage of tightly packing the wound with ribbon gauze is that the dressing may well act as a bung preventing free discharge from the cavity and dressing material may actually be lost in the cavity. The object of dressing this type of wound is not to pack the cavity, but to break down any granulation tissue at the skin edge and prevent the edges becoming adherent by loosely packing the orifice. If this is done the wound will heal up by granulation from the bottom.

Very deep wounds such as an empyema cavity are particularly liable to give problems in healing because the cavity is large and the sinus opening relatively small. Narrowing of the sinus opening and poor drainage are very likely to occur. A tube drain prevents the sinus closing and provides excellent drainage. As the cavity closes, the tube is progressively withdrawn — the situation being monitored by a series of sinograms.

FISTULAE

As already explained a fistula is a track connecting two epithelial surfaces. Many types of fistulae involving various different organs can occur in the body either as a result of congenital or acquired conditions. However, dealing with external wounds only, the fistulae under discussion are those between a viscus and the skin. The viscus involved may be any part of the gastrointestinal or genitourinary tract.

Some fistulae are created by a planned surgical procedure and examples are ileostomy, colostomy, nephrostomy and suprapubic catheterisation. Others develop spontaneously and unexpectedly either as the result of a disease process or, more commonly, following surgery. The common diseases causing fistulation are inflammatory conditions, especially Crohn's disease and malignancy. In fact, fistulae occur most commonly, not from some disease process, but as the unexpected and unintended result of surgery. The fistula is usually due to the breakdown of an anastomosis, but may also occur from inadvertent damage to a viscus from a suction drain or a loop of bowel being trapped between deep tension sutures.

The fistula is discovered when fluid or pus discharges either from a drain or through the wound. *Examination of the fistula fluid* will in most cases enable the diagnosis of the site of the fistula and the direction of appropriate treatment.

Fluid from a gastric fistula is very variable, sometimes consisting of watery gastric juice which, perhaps, contains flecks of altered blood. It may be bile-stained or contain tea, fruit juices or whatever the patient has recently drunk. A comparison with the aspirate from a nasogastric tube will usually provide the answer. The diagnosis can be confirmed by testing the discharge with Litmus paper, by inserting some methylene blue into the stomach or by gastrograffin meal. A bile-stained discharge may have come from the biliary tree, stomach or duodenum. Excoriation of the skin around the fistula strongly suggests involvement of the small bowel or pancreas. Pancreatic fluid is colourless. Yellowy orange fluid suggests small bowel origin. A faecal fistula with the large bowel commonly presents with a purulent discharge from the drainage tube which later becomes faecal. Large quantities of serous fluid draining from the abdomen or pelvis suggest a urinary fistula. Measurement of the urea content and comparison with the serum level is helpful in confirming the diagnosis. Special radiological investigations are often necessary to determine the site of the fistula, although in most cases this can be inferred from a knowledge of the operation performed.

The treatment of fistulae

There are three aspects to the treatment of fistulae.

1 Care of the skin
2 Nutritional support
3 Surgery

A discussion in order of their importance follows:

Care of the skin

This is the first consideration. If not dealt with promptly the skin around the fistula may become excoriated and sore within an hour or so and present considerable problems in management.

If large quantities of fluid are being produced from a fistula, this must be efficiently collected by an appropriate drain or appliance so that the patient is kept dry and comfortable. It is most important to measure the volume of the discharge from the fistula so that the fluid loss is known and can be replaced. In some cases this may amount to as much as 2 litres a day. If the volume lost is not accurately recorded and replaced the patient may become dangerously fluid and electrolyte depleted. A knowledge of the fluid loss is also the most reliable guide as to whether or not the fistula is healing.

If a drain is already *in situ*, simply connecting this to a bedside urine drainage bag may suffice. However, sooner or later fluid will begin to leak around the tube and it is then best to cut the end off so that it drains into a bag which is placed over the whole lot. If the fistula output is high, there must be continuous drainage of the bag otherwise it will become dislodged by the weight of its contents. This situation is best managed using a drainage stoma bag emptying through a drainage tube attached to its tapered end. The problem of making a bag stick to sore, excoriated skin has been largely overcome by the use of Stomahesive® or other adhesive materials. Stomahesive is a compressed wafer of gelatin, pectin and methyl cellulose which has the property of sticking to moist surfaces. Its use has revolutionised the management of these difficult problems and made obsolete earlier methods, such as nursing the patient face down on a split bed, sump suction and the use of aluminium paste.

There are still, however, some patients whose fistulae are extremely difficult to

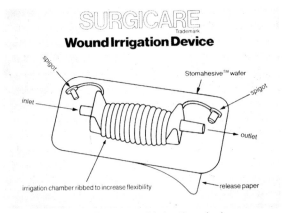

Fig 9.6 The wound irrigation device.

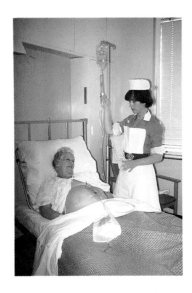

manage because of their site. If this is related to a fold, a depression or a bony prominence, such as the rib cage or iliac crest, movement is likely to dislodge the appliance. Any depression will need to be built up and cracks and grooves filled in with Karaya gum paste before the Stomahesive is applied.

A fistula arising from the centre of a dehisced wound presents one of the greatest challenges in nursing and requires the help and expertise of a trained Stomacare Nurse. If the wound is reasonably small and not too wide, the situation is most easily managed with a wound irrigation device. This consists of an adhesive rim of Stomahesive fused to a transparent plastic cover with entry and exit ports to permit irrigation and drainage of fluid from the fistula (Fig 9.6). The device is greatly appreciated by patients and staff as it does away with smell and frequent dressings, as well as keeping the surrounding skin healthy. It may not need to be changed for several days. Figure 9.7 illustrates the device being successfully used in a patient with wound breakdown and a pancreatic fistula. The wound irrigation device is not suitable for patients with fistulae when there is extensive wound breakdown as in Fig 9.8. Some form of sump suction is required, in this case provided by a Shirley drain, to convey the fistula fluid away from the wound. Pieces of Stomahesive are then applied to the wound edges and any gaps, grooves or depressions filled in with

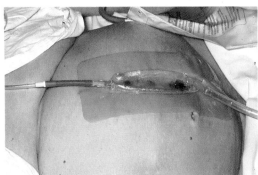

Fig 9.7 Wound breakdown and pancreatic fistula following drainage of a pancreatic abscess — successfully managed with wound irrigation device.

Karaya gum paste. The whole area is then covered with Op-site or Steridrape®, bringing the drainage tubes through a hole made in the centre and reinforcing the edges with Micropore.®

Sump suction drainage is never totally efficient and there are occasions when the tubing blocks or the output is too fast for the drain to cope. It is, therefore, almost always necessary to reduce fistula drainage as much as possible by restricting oral fluids. Cimetidine may also be helpful in reducing the secretion of gastrointestinal juices.

Maintaining nutrition
Normal healing is dependent on a patient's

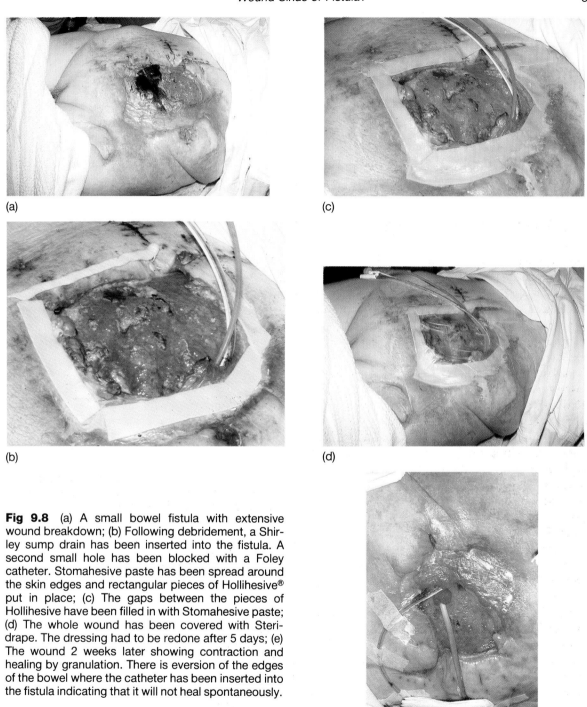

Fig 9.8 (a) A small bowel fistula with extensive wound breakdown; (b) Following debridement, a Shirley sump drain has been inserted into the fistula. A second small hole has been blocked with a Foley catheter. Stomahesive paste has been spread around the skin edges and rectangular pieces of Hollihesive® put in place; (c) The gaps between the pieces of Hollihesive have been filled in with Stomahesive paste; (d) The whole wound has been covered with Steri-drape. The dressing had to be redone after 5 days; (e) The wound 2 weeks later showing contraction and healing by granulation. There is eversion of the edges of the bowel where the catheter has been inserted into the fistula indicating that it will not heal spontaneously.

nutritional status. The majority of patients with gastrointestinal fistulae have undergone recent surgery and are likely to be malnourished.

Enteral nutrition should be used wherever possible, but with a high fistula parenteral feeding is essential.

Surgery

It is important to realise that most fistulae will close spontaneously and, therefore, a policy of conservative management should be adopted in most cases. There are, however, certain situations where healing is unlikely to occur and these are listed below.

1   In the presence of distal obstruction.
2   Where there is carcinoma at the site of the fistula.
3   When epithelisation of the fistulous track has occurred.
4   In the case of injury or disruption of an anastomosis where the bowel mucosa has become everted. (This can only be determined at operation.)
5   In Crohn's disease (but not always).

It is sometimes a great temptation for a surgeon to reopen a patient with a fistula in an attempt to close it. In the presence of sepsis and malnutrition such a course is unlikely to lead to success and may well end in disaster. With nutritional support, control of sepsis and time, most fistulae will heal. Those that do not should be operated on only when the patient has been made as fit as possible and the nutritional state is normal.

Chapter 10

Tetanus and Antibiotic Prophylaxis

Stephen Westaby

TETANUS

Clostridium tetani is an anaerobic bacillus found in cultivated soil and in the gut of man and animals. Tetanus is a rare disease in Western countries, but remains an important cause of mortality in underdeveloped countries where standards of hygiene and primary wound care are lower. Neonatal tetanus is an important cause of infant death in regions where the practice of applying cow dung to the umbilical stump persists.

The clinical features of tetanus are the result of a potent neurotoxin 'tetanospasmin' produced by the bacillus. This is a high molecular weight protein avidly taken up by the gangliosides of the central nervous system and it has been estimated that 1 kg of tetanospasmin would be sufficient to kill the population of the whole world. From the site of the wound the toxin travels directly up the motor network of the peripheral nerves to the spinal cord and medulla. In the anterior horn of the spinal cord the toxin is taken up by the presynaptic terminals of inhibitory spinal neurons preventing release of inhibitory spinal transmitters. This results in excessive discharge from motor nerves that is characteristic of tetanus. There is no effect on the sensory system, cerebral cortex or medulla, but removal of sympathetic

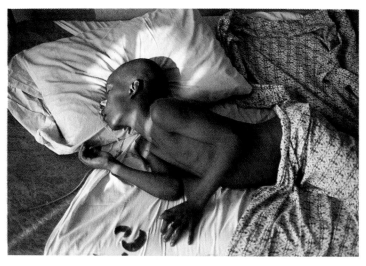

Fig 10.1 Extensor spasm in a child with tetanus.

inhibition in the lateral horn of the spinal cord accounts for the excessive sympathetic activity seen in severe tetanus. Because transit of toxin occurs slowly, the first effects are seen in muscle groups with short motor neurons; the head and neck muscles followed by the trunk and lastly the limb muscles.

Trismus and dysphagia are the initial features in most cases, hence the colloquial name 'lockjaw'. The muscular hypertonicity then spreads to the neck, back, abdomen and limbs. Once seen the clinical signs are characteristic. If the disease is severe, muscular spasms of increasing frequency and duration are superimposed on the hypertonicity resulting in crush fractures of the vertebrae and death from respiratory failure and exhaustion. The patient's initial complaint is of spasm of the facial muscles producing the classic 'Risus sardonicus', then rigidity of the neck, back and abdomen. Variations may occur such as cephalic tetanus, when a wound around the head or neck is followed by cranial nerve palsies, usually unilateral facial palsy and sometimes weakness of the extraoccular muscles with diplopia. In local tetanus there is hypertonicity of the muscles in the region of the wound. Both variations usually progress to generalised tetanus.

Any wound may be a portal of entry though, in practice, a wound can be identified in only 60% of cases. Deep penetrating injuries with a focus of necrotic tissue and infection are particularly at risk. Foreign bodies such as a splinter, thorns, road gravel or glass increase the likelihood of infection though clean surgical wounds have also been implicated. The incubation period varies between 3–21 days and tends to be shorter in severe cases. The interval between the first symptom and first spasm varies from less than 24 hours to over 10 days and the shorter the period the worse the attack. Severity varies from mild trismus and muscle stiffness to a rapidly progressive illness ending in agonising death within 48 hours. Though there is considerable variation in incubation period and period of onset, the duration of the established illness is uniform with

progression of severity during the first week, plateau during the second and improvement in the third if death does not intervene. In the recovery phase, stiffness may persist for several weeks especially in the calf muscles and residual cranial nerve palsies occur in those presenting with cephalic tetanus lasting for 2–3 weeks. Reported mortality rates vary widely from nil to over 100% and results from intensive care units in Western countries, where experience of the disease is limited, are not always better than those obtained by conservative treatment in countries such as India where vast numbers of cases are treated.

PROPHYLAXIS

Active immunisation of the entire population could virtually eliminate tetanus. The first major step came in the 1890s with the introduction of horse derived tetanus antitoxin for passive immunisation (the administration of preformed antibodies). The next advance was the development of a procedure for active immunisation (the induction of antibodies within the host) following the introduction of tetanus toxoid in the 1920s. The arrival of penicillin provided a means of complementing the immediate protection provided by the antitoxin, though the efficacy of antibiotics in the prevention of tetanus is debatable.

Immunisation with absorbed tetanus toxoid is extremely effective and safe. Ideally everyone, regardless of age, should have an adequate level of circulating antibodies to tetanus and thus be immune to the disease. Man does not develop natural immunity; therefore, to achieve the state of full immunity and thus be protected should a wound be sustained, a programme of active immunisation with tetanus vaccine must be carried out. A basic course consists of 3 spaced doses with 6 weeks between the first and second and 6 months between the second and third. A routine booster dose should follow at 10-year intervals. Reactions to toxoid are rare, usually minor and more likely if frequent booster doses are given. Adequate antibody levels are rarely attained following the first dose of toxoid and effective protection is not usually acquired until after the second dose. A strategy for prophylaxis is, therefore, needed in the wounded, non-immunised patient and for those in whom immunisation is incomplete. Such a scheme is shown in Fig 10.2.

Firstly, all wounds should receive appropriate surgical toilet, cleansing the area of dirt, devitalised tissue and contaminated organisms. However, many tetanus contaminated wounds are very minor and more serious wounds may show no sign or symptom of infection. Antibiotics such as penicillin and tetracycline have been shown to be effective against vegetative tetanus bacilli, but, clearly, have no effect against toxin and may not achieve antibacterial levels in the presence of poor local blood supply. Both wound debridement and antibiotics have played an important part in reducing the incidence of tetanus, but cannot be relied upon to prevent it. Pas-

sive immunisation with antitetanus serum at the time of wounding is very effective. Recently, there has been an increasing awareness of the problems associated with the use of horse derived antitoxin, principally a high incidence of adverse reactions in up to 25% of patients. Fatal anaphylactic shock is estimated to occur at the rate of 1 in 200 000 injections, and adrenaline injection should be available. A further disadvantage is the lack of efficacy of horse antitoxin in patients already sensitised. Immune globulin of human origin has fewer disadvantages, its only contraindication being a history of anaphylaxis resulting from previous administration of human gamma globulin. An advantage is that it is a natural human protein eliminated very slowly and consequently maintaining an effective level of protection for up to 4 weeks. It provides immediate protection against circulating tetanus toxin. The purified immunoglobulin is obtained from the sera of healthy human donors known to have high levels of tetanus antitoxin follow-

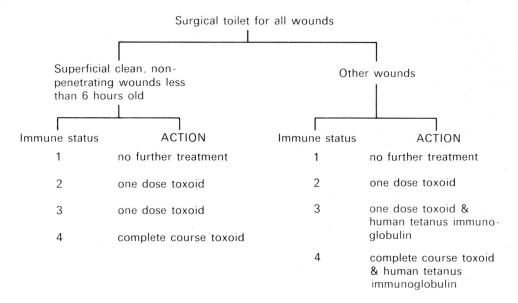

Categories of immune status

1 Previous complete course of toxoid or a booster dose within last 5 years.
2 Previous complete course of toxoid or a booster dose between 5 and 10 years ago.
3 Previous complete course of toxoid or a booster dose 10 years ago.
4 No complete course of toxoid or immune status unknown.

Fig 10.2 Tetanus prophylaxis.

ing active immunisation with tetanus vaccine. Each vial contains 250 iu of antitoxin in 1.0 ml solution and is given by intramuscular injection. A prophylactic active immunisation schedule should follow. Details of the treatment of established tetanus will not be discussed and are available elsewhere. Specific control of the organism and toxin are achieved by administration of human antitetatnus serum (intramuscularly, intravenously or intrathecally) and benzyll penicillin. When a wound can be identified, it should be widely excised to healthy tissue, irrigated with hydrogen peroxide and left open. It may be left to granulate or closed by suture or graft some days later. Symptomatic treatment with sedation and muscle relaxants or neuromuscular blockade with artificial ventilation are required.

Selection of patients or wounds requiring antibiotic prophylaxis

There are two major considerations in the discussion of when to employ antibiotic prophylaxis. Firstly, is a particular patient especially at risk from infection by virtue of a separate problem at the time of wounding or surgery? Secondly, is a type of wound or operation likely to place a normal patient at risk from a dangerous infection? These categories will be considered separately.

The susceptible patient
The concept that certain illnesses predispose to infection after wounding or surgical operations is not new, though the ability to identify such patients and treat them prophylactically belongs to the last two decades. Such condi-

Table 1
CONDITIONS PREDISPOSING TO INFECTION

Clinical	Investigational
Diabetes	Anaemia
Drugs	Hypoalbumenaemia
Malnutrition	Abnormal immunoglobulins
Malignancy	Lymphopenia
Alcoholism	Anergy

tions basically alter the interplay between bacterial invasion and host defences; some are clinically apparent, others only revealed by informed investigation (Table 1).

It is well recognised that the diabetic is prone to sepsis. Though it remains unclear as to how the severity of diabetes and its treatment at the time of wounding affects the likelihood of sepsis, it is important to maintain optimum control. Some drugs, especially steroids, cytotoxics and immunosupressive agents, result in poor healing and inability to combat infection. Malnutrition further contributes to risk, especially protein depletion. Definition of protein malnutrition poses a problem, but the simplest estimates are weight loss and the number of protein meals the patient has per week. Thus a 5 kg loss over a recent 3-month period or a consumption of meat, chicken or fish less than five times per week are a reasonable estimate for likelihood of malnutrition. Serum albumen or transferrin levels and total body potassium provide confirmatory evidence. The presence of malignant disease especially when widespread and metastatic predisposes to infections, but past malignant disease which has been removed or controlled is probably not of importance. Similarly, alcoholism is associated with protein malnutrition and alcoholic liver disease results in hypoalbumenaemia. The amount of alcohol drunk is the most significant factor. Eight or more alcoholic drinks per day for 10 years or more constitutes an important risk.

There are a number of investigations which may be used as markers for risk of sepsis after surgery and are useful in the presence of clinical evidence of risk. Uncorrected anaemia with haemoglobin of less than 10 g in females and less than 12 g in males and reduced serum albumen levels are associated with increased likelihood of sepsis. Lymphopenia with a decrease in the total number of lymphocytes to 1500/ml or less is an important marker of immune incompetence. Agammaglobulinaemias are associated with recurrent infections, including postoperative infections, but rarely pose problems in surgery. Relatively minimal alterations of immunoglobulin levels, often associated with malnutrition or malignant disease, have been associated with sepsis after elective operations.

Delayed hypersensitivity skin tests have been shown to be a practical indicator of surgical sepsis. Reaction to the antigens of mumps, trichophyton, streptokinase, tuberculin and candida when considered in the light of clinical risk factors (such as malnutrition) have been found to be highly predictive of postoperative sepsis. The antigens are injected intradermally and read after 48 hours. A positive response is recorded if there is inflammation of greater than 6 × 6 mm. Normal adults will have two or more positive in this battery of tests. Thus one positive response only indicates abnormality in immunological response and no positive response indicates specific abnormality called anergy. High risk patients can also be shown to have poor neutrophil killing of staphylococci, but the relationship of this test to other clinical and simpler investigational risk factors has not so far been determined.

In practical terms, it seems realistic to identify the surgical patient at risk by eliciting a history of diabetes, malnutrition, malignant disease, chronic alcoholism or the use of immuno-suppressive drugs. Reinforcement by haemoglobin estimation, serum proteins and total lymphocyte count is relatively inexpensive enough to be employed routinely. In the near future anergy and neutrophil killing of bacteria may be of discriminatory value.

Having identified those patients at risk, prophylactic antibiotics still should not be used on a routine basis, but considered on the grounds of bacterial contamination. Most traumatic wounds are heavily contaminated and in a susceptible patient appropriate prophylaxis in the form of a wide spectrum antibiotic is given when first seen, though antibiotics are not a substitute for wound toilet or debridement. For elective or emergency surgery, it has long been recognised that certain aspects of the procedure itself contribute to the likelihood of sepsis. For example, obese patients are at risk because of increased area of contamination. Such factors are considered in the following section.

One further group of patients requiring regular antibiotic prophylaxis are those with congenital or acquired heart disease, vascular implants or prosthetic heart valves, who are at risk from bacterial endocarditis. Events which place such patients at risk include dental treatment, minor wounds or infected abrasions, urinary manipulations and passage of intravenous catheters. Endocarditis is a lethal condition, particularly when unrecognised in its early stages or involving valve prostheses or vascular grafts. Well established guidelines for prophylaxis are available elsewhere.

Wounds and surgical procedures which require antibiotic prophylaxis

Bacterial contamination is an important determinant of infection after trauma or elective surgery. Additional factors are the surface area of the open wound and the duration of exposure to the atmosphere (length of operation). In practice, operations may be considered clean or contaminated and either small and simple or large and complicated. Clean operations may be defined as those where there is no acute inflammation. Infection during these circumstances is the consequence of innocculation of bacteria into the wound by breach of surgical technique. Clean procedures constitute the bulk of general operations such as herniorrhaphy, breast and endocrine surgery. The majority of head and neck surgery may be classified clean, so long as the gastrointestinal and respiratory tracts are not opened. Other specialities with a high incidence of clean operations include ENT, neuro, plastic, cardiac, orthopaedic and peripheral vascular surgery. Apart from peripheral vascular surgery, where tissue ischaemia predisposes to infection, the sepsis rate in clean surgery is less than 2%. Risk increases at the extremes of life, in patients who have been in hospital for a long time or are nasal staphylococcal carriers and with increasing duration of operation. The predominant cause of clean wound infection is *Staphylococcus aureus*.

As previously discussed in Chapter 8 for analysis of risk, surgical procedures may be classified into four types. Risk increases from 1–4.

1 Small clean operations (herniorrhaphy, mastectomy, thyroidectomy)
2 Large clean operations (cardiac surgery, hip replacement, etc)
3 Small contaminated operations (appendectomy, choleocystectomy, etc)
4 Large contaminated operations (colorectal surgery, thoracotomy for oesophageal perforation etc).

Wherever a hollow viscus containing bacteria is opened, there is considerable risk of sepsis. In general, antibiotic cover is used only where there is a high risk of sepsis or where sepsis, though rare, is associated with life-threatening consequences. In addition, it is preferable to recommend antibiotic prophylaxis only when its value has been analysed. The term prophylaxis is only applied when there has been no preoperative contamination or established infection and for this reason antibiotics used for traumatic wounds and acute inflammatory disease, such as appendicitis, cannot strictly be considered prophylactic. In general, prophylaxis is not required for small clean operations or the majority of large clean, or small contaminated procedures, though metronidazole has proven so effective in the control of infection after appendectomy that this is now used routinely. Large contaminated procedures benefit from well planned antibiotic prophylaxis and the antibiotic employed is tailored to the expected contaminant.

Life-threatening consequences associated with operations other than large contaminated procedures include infection in arterial grafts or prosthetic heart valves, infected orthopaedic implants and neurosurgical shunts. The incidence of infection in implant surgery varies from centre to centre, but the consequences are invariably disasterous. Prosthetic joint replacement may be associated with deep wound sepsis in 0.6 — 2.1% of patients. Patients usually develop pain at the site, due to chronic osteomyelitis. Infected neurosurgical shunts for hydrocephalus result in ventriculitis or meningitis. Sepsis in cardiovascular surgery is even more serious. Prosthetic valve endocarditis occurs in less than 1% of patients, but carries a mortality approaching 50%. Infection of a peripheral vascular graft occurs in less than 2% of patients, usually when the groin has been exposed. The mortality of graft sepsis is more than 25% and limb amputation is required in half of the patients.

Most infections around implants are from low grade pathogens such as *Staphylococcus epidermidis*, micrococcus and *Serratia*. *Staphylococcus aureus* is still the predominant pathogen in joint replacement. Antibiotic prophylaxis is, therefore, strongly recommended in the above groups and is of proven value in patients with bacteruria requiring urological operations and in patients having vaginal or abdominal hysterectomy. They should be used prior to emergency biliary operations and in elective biliary operations in patients over 70, those who are jaundiced or who are known to have stones or strictures in the bile duct. In general, patients undergoing surgery on the upper gastrointestinal tract do not require antibiotics in the absence of malignant disease. Tumours encourage the growth of abnormal flora however, and usually warrant antibiotic cover since patients with extensive malignant disease have greater susceptibility. This also applies to patients with bronchogenic carcinoma undergoing thoracotomy for lung resection.

The highest incidence of postoperative sepsis occurs in patients undergoing colorectal surgery. Not only is infection of the abdominal or perineal wound a frequent complication, but pelvic abscess or septicaemia is also common and dangerous. The principal pathogenic organisms are anaerobic bacteria such as *Bacteroides*, *Clostridia*, and anaerobic streptococci, and aerobic species including *Escherichia coli*, *Proteus*, *Klebsiella* and *Pseudomonas*.

It should be emphasised that antibiotic prophylaxis is not a substitute for poor surgical technique. Notably, inadequate haemostasis, strangulating sutures, inabsorbable materials and open drains contribute to the likelihood of sepsis.

The key to prevention of infection is to obtain a high dose of antibiotic in the tissues and circulation at the time at which bacteria will be innocculated into the operation site. The antibiotic should preferably be bactericidal. Routes for administrating antimicrobial prophylaxis include:

1 oral agents which may be used with preoperative bowel preparation;
2 topical agents which can be injected into the peritoneal cavity or wound;
3 systemic prophylaxis.

There is no doubt that systemic administration by intravenous injection just prior to operation is the best course. This serves to eliminate endogenous organisms as they are released into the tissue. A single dose is probably effective, though a second may be given shortly after the procedure. Systemic injection provides predictable serum levels. Oral agents may increase the risk of bacterial resistance or allow overgrowth of staphylococci or yeasts and have been implicated as a cause of pseudomembranous colitis. Topical agents have not been shown to have any value in elective procedures and whereas antibiotics placed into the wound may prevent sepsis locally, they do not protect against intra-abdominal abscess or septicaemia.

Chapter 11

Treatment of Wounds in the Accident and Emergency Department

Stephen Westaby and Alison Thorn

The majority of wounds treated in the Accident and Emergency unit are minor, but should not be underestimated. Most result from accidents at work, in the home or during recreational activities. The remainder are due to road traffic accidents, physical assault or animal bites. The accident department must be capable of providing a 24-hour service and of handling a number of patients simultaneously. The patients themselves frequently present additional difficulties. In the evening many are drunk, aggressive and either unable or unwilling to give a satisfactory clinical history. Others attempt suicide, mutilate themselves or attempt to disguise an assault by family or friends. Their motives should be determined when possible so that further support may follow treatment of their physical wounds. Frightened children must be handled with patience and sympathy both by medical and nursing staff. Their parents are usually anxious and protective, but their wishes should be respected and intended treatment discussed in advance.

Though most abrasions; superficial lacerations and minor burns heal promptly without or in spite of active intervention, great care must be taken to assess such wounds accurately and carefully. Undetected fractures or foreign bodies, unrevealed deep penetration of fascial spaces or nerve injury may lead to serious late medical or legal problems. Well meaning but innappropriate suture of dirty lacerations, unnecessarily restrictive splints or dressings and indiscriminate prescription of antibiotics are an everyday feature of most accident departments. Few errors result in serious debility, but many result in prolongation of recovery and much needless expense. In Britain the policies for medical staffing of accident departments are partly responsible in that most casualty officers are recently qualified and without experience of wound care, orthopaedics or major trauma. Frequently there is little or no senior supervision and considerable reliance on guidance from experienced nursing staff. With knowledge of the basic principles of wound care many mistakes may be avoided. This chapter outlines certain policies relevant to the accident department and discusses the range of wounds commonly encountered.

TRIAGE

The work load is variable and clearly, unless the staffing is excessive for normal requirements, it will on occasion be insufficient. Triage is the assessment of priorities in a busy situation. It is more usual to discuss triage in relation to major accidents with multiple casualties. Those with minor wounds or irrecoverably major injuries are set aside, whilst those with more serious but treatable wounds are salvaged. Priorities are decided by a senior member of the medical team. In the context of a busy accident department under pressure from large numbers of 'walking wounded', it is necessary to deploy an experienced nurse or casualty officer to perform a similar role. It is important that the receptionist is eliminated from this role, which requires medical knowledge, confidence, authority and determination. Sundry medical problems such as earache, skin rashes, toothache, coughs and colds must be refused admittance and more serious medical and surgical emergencies referred directly to the appropriate specialists. Those units which fail to exercise this function soon become ineffective.

One of the most important decisions to be made by the casualty officer is whether to treat the wounded patient personally or seek advice from others. This depends both upon experience and the time and facilities required to treat the wound itself. In general, the following types of wound should be seen by a specialist:

1 Penetrating wounds of the chest or abdomen
2 Penetrating wounds of the brain or spinal cord
3 Compound factures, however small
4 Burns with any systemic disturbance
5 Lacerations with major vascular, nerve or tendon involvement
6 Facial wounds associated with faciomaxillary fractures
7 Wounds of the eye
8 Wounds with potential medico-legal or forensic importance
9 Wounds with foreign bodies requiring surgical intervention for removal
10 Wounds associated with blunt internal injuries.

The necessity for referral does not relate to the competence of the casualty officer, but to the requirement for specialised facilities and long-term follow up. Such patients must be transferred promptly after assessment and first aid. There should be no interference with the wound itself apart from cleansing and application of a protective dressing.

Practical wound care by nursing staff also requires consideration. It is common for trained nurses to suture uncomplicated lacerations, though nursing policy differs widely. In the United States 'surgical technicians' and nurse practitioners are trained in wound care and taught suturing techniques. They become at least as skilled as most surgeons in a limited and well defined area of therapy. This approach is cost effective by releasing medical staff from time-consuming repetitive work. It is important that every wound is carefully assessed by the doctor who then directs, but does not have to carry out, the prescribed treatment. If British nurses are to adopt a similar role in the accident department, they should receive formal training and recognition. Most enjoy this additional responsibility and participation in patient care.

INITIAL ASSESSMENT AND FIRST AID

A friendly and reassuring reception is an important prelude to further treatment. Gaining the confidence of a child and its parents at an early stage greatly facilitates manipulation of the wound itself when the time comes. Long waits with other injured or complaining patients is undesirable. Frequently, the wound will have been covered immediately to stem bleeding and the patient may not have seen or come to terms with his injury. Reassurance is vital, since all patients are apprehensive and even the toughest male is not immune to fainting at the sight of his own blood.

A careful clinical history should be fully documented in hospital records for each case. Industrial compensation, criminal prosecution or a legal suit for malpractice may depend on the evidence from such notes, often in the most unexpected circumstances. The possibility and nature of a foreign body is questioned. The extent of the wound and potential degree of contamination is assessed with the knowledge of the mechanism of injury. The size of the wound is not always indicative of its seriousness. A stab wound may initially appear as a small skin laceration though the underlying damage to muscle, tendon, nerve or blood vessels may be extensive. Amount of blood loss should be assessed by examination of blood-soaked clothing or previously discarded dressings, since the vital signs are a poor predictor of volume of haemorrhage. The status of tetanus prophylaxis is sought. If such information cannot be obtained from the patient, accompanying personnel should be questioned. Whilst the history is documented, the nurse should expose the wound. Conversation distracts the patient's interest temporarily.

In the absence of major vascular injury bleeding has usually stopped by a process of retraction and thrombosis of the smaller vessels. Persistent haemorrhage is controlled by local pressure, if necessary whilst the patient is sedated. The physiological response to blood loss generates anxiety by cathacholamine release and loss of 1000 ml or more requires prompt replacement with an appropriate volume expander. Only then will the patient manage to relax and cooperate. Sedation and pain relief are best given together, for instance by morphine injection. Consideration must be given to the necessity for general anaesthesia, since the anaesthetist will not appreciate a recent cup of tea or oral analgesics taken with water.

Removal of clothing from the area may prove difficult and there should be no hesitation in cutting them away if necessary. This should be done as soon as possible, since clothes carry a wealth of bacteria and bacterial spores. Inevitably all traumatic wounds are contaminated. Burns are initially self sterilising, but rapidly contaminated shortly afterwards. Foreign bodies drive clothing or dirt deep into the tissues and are particularly a

haven for anaerobic organisms such as *Cl. tetani* or *Cl. welchii* (gas gangrene). Industrial or farming wounds are usually impregnated with oil, grit, soil or metal particles.

The first step in wound toilet is to clean the surroundings as effectively as possible before a full assessment of damage is made. This is usually performed by firm rubbing of the area with antiseptic soaked swabs or cotton wool. Particles of grit and other foreign materials are picked out with forceps. The principles of surgical asepsis as used in the operating theatre strictly speaking do not apply at this stage. Swabs are held in forceps or clean fingers so as not to introduce further bacteria or foreign material. One exception to this is in the treatment of burns, which are initially clean, and strict asepsis techniques should be observed. The two most commonly applied antiseptics are providone iodine and chlorhexidine, both of which are available as alcoholic and aqueous solutions (Table 1).

Table 1
EFFECTIVE ANTISEPTIC SOLUTIONS

Alcoholic	0.5% chlorhexidine in 70% alcohol
	Providone iodine (1% available I_2) in 30% alcohol, 70% ethanol
Aqueous	0.5% chlorhexidine
	Providone iodine (1% available I_2)

Alcoholic solutions are particularly effective in skin cleansing, but because of their caustic nature are best avoided in the wound itself. Aqueous solutions are less rapidly bactericidal in the presence of dirt or grease, but do not damage the cells exposed in the depth of the wound and are, therefore, preferable for exposed tissue. If disturbance of blood clot during cleaning causes renewed bleeding, haemostasis is achieved by application of a clean pressure dressing or suture ligation.

Once clean and dry, the extent of damage to the skin, soft tissues and vital structures (nerve, blood vessels, bone, tendon, etc) can be properly determined.

DECISION MAKING AND FURTHER TREATMENT

Many superficial lacerations, abrasions and minor burns require little more than cleansing and an occlusive dressing pending re-epithelisation of the area which occurs rapidly over the next few days. Tetanus prophylaxis is given when appropriate and the patient discharged.

Deeper lacerations require careful examination to exclude penetration and introduction of bacteria into underlying fascial spaces (especially in the hand), Lacerations caused by glass should be examined radiologically for splinters if there is the slightest suspicion of retained material (Fig 11.1). The decision to

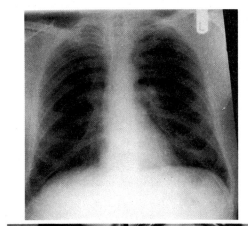

(a)

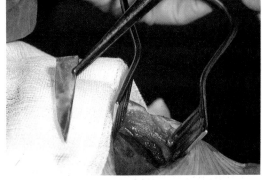

(b)

Fig 11.1 (a) Chest x-ray showing retained fragment of glass within the pleural cavity of a patient who fell through a greenhouse roof. A large fragment had previously been removed from the chest wall and the man sent home. (b) Surgical removal of the retained fragment 1 week later.

close a wound depends on the adequacy of wound toilet. Cleanly incised lacerations without foreign bodies can be safely closed by sutures or tapes. Deep wounds may require absorbable synthetic or Catgut sutures to fascia or muscle layers. Cut tendons or nerves may be repaired primarily if the surgeon is sure that potential bacterial contaminants have been eliminated and that wound closure is safe. Such repairs should be performed in the operating theatre using magnification and appropriate suture materials. Wounds contaminated by soil or heavily impregnated with dust or grit are best left open covered by clean dressings. The process of wound contraction and granulation (healing by secondary intention) will result in an acceptable scar and the considerable risk of serious wound sepsis is eliminated. Damaged nerves and tendons are then repaired at a later stage when the wound has healed without sepsis. Small areas of skin loss are usually left to granulate, though clean avulsion injuries of the fingers are best dealt with by skin grafting. Larger areas of skin loss require skin grafting by a plastic surgeon. Dressings should protect the wound, but be kept to a minimum so as not to disturb movement of the part. Patients must be given clear instructions on future care of their wound and be advised if and when to attend for further dressings, removal of sutures or other treatment. Most after-care can be dealt with by the general practitioner or district nurse. Some accident departments have a separate follow-up clinic, but this should not interfere with the treatment of acute injuries.

ANAESTHESIA AND ANALGESIA

The majority of minor wounds need no anaesthetic for cleansing or dressing, though some anxious patients appreciate an oral sedative. Extensive abrasions with impregnation of dirt or grit and some burns are best cleaned and debrided under general anaesthetic using a scrubbing brush. Failure to clean them adequately by denying general anaesthetic results in a disfiguring tatoo effect.

Anaesthesia for closure of lacerations depends on their extent and the technique to be used. Most cleanly incised superficial lacerations can be closed satisfactorily and painlessly with skin tapes and sutures should be avoided wherever possible. Deeper lacerations benefit from closure of underlying tissue layers by suturing. Satisfactory anaesthesia is then desirable not only for the patient's pain relief but also to provide cooperation and prevent movement during the procedure. Up to three simple sutures can reasonably be performed quickly without local anaesthesia for wounds up to 5 cm in length in adults and some older children. Lignocaine injection usually necessitates more than one skin prick and the acidic nature of the drug gives discomfort or pain for many patients. Larger lacerations, those with irregular contours requiring detailed work, and deep wounds requiring subcutaneous sutures should be liberally anaesthetised with lignocaine. The systemic effects of lignocaine must not be forgotten and the dosage should be monitored. 10 ml of 1% solution without adrenaline is usually adequate. Lignocaine with adrenaline should never be used for 'ring' nerve blockade of digits, since the swelling and vasoconstriction in combination may cause ischaemic necrosis. Lignocaine 0.5% can be used for more extensive areas in combination with an intramuscular opiate analgesic. Extensive facial injuries caused by windscreen glass need careful wound toilet to eliminate foreign bodies and plastic surgical repair under general anaesthesia. They are often associated with injury to the eye.

Children must be considered separately and general anaesthesia used much more frequently. The necessity to use sutures rather than tapes must be justified. One or two sutures may be attempted using ethylchloride spray though this has little effect. Children hate needles and the sight of local anaesthetic needles may cause havoc for subsequent suturing. It is much kinder to perform the repair expeditiously under a short general anaesthetic, thus sparing the child, parent and doctor from a harrowing experience. It is very diffi-

cult to know whether to allow the parent to stay with the child if local anaesthetic is used. Some are very good with a calming influence, others fall about and transmit anxiety.

COMMON WOUNDS ON A REGIONAL BASIS

Wounds to the head and face

These are particularly common in all age groups since the area is continually exposed and vulnerable. Infants, as they begin to crawl and walk, are constantly knocking into furniture and lacerations from such injuries are common. They are usually minor and require only cleaning and taping for closure. With any head wound, the risk of greater damage must be considered and careful neurological assessment is essential. The elderly are also prone to falls as they become infirm and scalp lacerations are common. These tend to be more extensive cuts, because of the lack of elasticity and the papery thin texture of the skin. The area surrounding scalp wounds should be shaved and cleaned and the wound carefully examined before sutures are inserted (Fig 11.2).

Sports injuries produce many facial and scalp wounds. The stud of a football boot may inflict deep and dirty scalp lacerations. Squash racquets or cricket balls commonly cause lacerations, particularly around the eyebrows

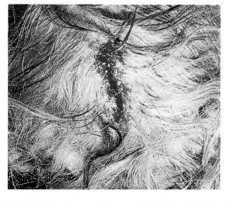

Fig 11.2   Scalp wound in an elderly lady following a fall.

and forehead. They are usually contaminated and adequate wound toilet is important.

Leaning over in an attempt to remove the radiator cap of an overheated engine is a common cause of facial scalds (Fig 11.3). Flash burns are mainly the result of industrial injuries, particularly in smelting processes and iron foundry work. Superficial burns and scalds, where the cutaneous peripheral nerve endings are not totally destroyed, are extremely painful. If burns or scalds are deep and extensive, admission to hospital will be necessary not only for local treatment of the wound, but also for the treatment of shock and correction of fluid balance. Superficial burns and scalds may look unsightly for a few days, but tend to heal rapidly and successfully.

Despite publicity and health education concerning the wearing of seat belts, an alarming number of severe facial lacerations and head injuries are seen following car accidents. Suturing these multiple lacerations is time-consuming and intricate and often best done by a plastic surgeon in a main operating theatre rather than in the A & E department. At first sight such injuries may seem alarming because of the brisk bleeding that always comes from scalp and facial wounds. With care these lacerations heal well, although scarring is inevitable.

Increasingly in this violent age facial

wounds are caused by assault from fists, boots, knives and other weapons. These wounds vary in their degree of severity, but tend to be contusions, lacerations and puncture wounds. The majority of scalp and facial wounds are left exposed after treatment. Few become infected and most heal quickly without problems.

Upper limb wounds

Wounds of the upper limb mostly involve the hands and digits and are by far the most common injuries seen in the A & E department. The variety is great but, again, the majority are fairly minor wounds which are easily treated and usually heal with few problems. Hand injuries should not be underestimated, since the simplest injury can cause great inconvenience and, if mismanaged, may lead to considerable disability and even permanent functional impairment.

Typical wounds to hands and fingers include crush injuries caused by trapping fingers in doors and cupboards. These can be severe with underlying bone injury and damage to the nail bed. Suturing may not be necessary or even possible and these wounds have to heal by granulation. Lacerations to the fingers from knives, tins, saws, chisels or other household objects and DIY tools are particularly common. Simple toilet and suturing is often all that is needed (Fig 11.4).

Industrial injuries may cause extensive damage if the hand is caught in moving machinery and traumatic amputation of the digits may result, requiring specialised surgery.

The incidence of wound infection in hand injuries is high because of contamination at the time of injury. Therefore, careful observation of these wounds is essential. Finger pulp, palmar and web space infections can be very troublesome and, if not properly treated, may result in necrosis and subsequent amputation.

Burns and scalds to the hand are common and must be dressed and checked regularly.

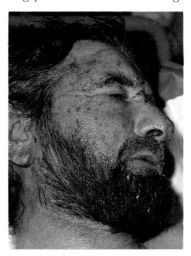

Fig 11.3

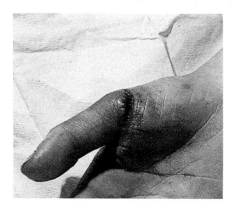

Fig 11.4 Laceration to thumb from whittling wood.

Encouragement should be given to the patient to continue active exercises of the fingers to avoid contractures. Electrical burns can be deep and grafting may be necessary.

Other injuries of the upper limbs include lacerations to the wrists with razor blades in attempted suicide cases. Several tentative lacerations are often made over the radial artery, but these are usually only superficial. Occasionally, tendons, nerves and arteries may be severed requiring meticulous repair by a skilled surgeon. Lacerations from glass can occur when an arm is pushed through a door or window and these wounds should be x-rayed to include overlooking any particles.

Abrasions to the prominences of the elbow or shoulder may occur following falls. These may be deep and contaminated and require thorough wound toilet. Dog and cat bites are another common feature and many can be surprisingly nasty. Fortunately, dog bites do not tend to become infected, but cat bites are more prone to infection and human bites are worst of all.

Wounds of the digits, hands and upper limb should be covered with a light but adequate dressing. Active movements of the affected part should be encouraged to minimise loss of function and to enable the patient to live as normally as possible. All wounds must be kept dry and this in itself can cause great inconvenience. For this reason, all injuries, however slight, must be taken seriously.

Management of open injuries to the hand

In the USA where power machinery is used extensively, 2 million disabling work injuries occur each year and 75% affect the hand. In Britain the problem is equally serious. Early and expert surgery is essential to minimise disability and shorten its duration. Skin damage is a dominant factor. A clean cut is the least serious, though damage to deep structures may occur even with small cuts. Irregular lacerations or degloving is more serious and crushed devitalised skin the worst of all. Examination must test active movements to assess tendon damage. Sensation is tested to assess possible nerve injury. X-rays are taken to detect fractures, dislocations or foreign bodies.

Whilst all acute hand injuries pass through the accident department, serious injuries require the combined skill of orthopaedic and plastic surgeons. Hand injuries may be classified as follows:

1 *Tidy injuries* — due to sharp agents such as glass or knives. The cuts are clean, may involve deeper structures and are common in children. Bony injury is uncommon. Primary repair is the usual form of treatment.

2 *Untidy injuries* — these are common in industry. The skin is ragged and there may be multiple fractures. It is essential to obtain skin coverage after excision of all devitalised tissue by whichever method is applicable — suture, skin grafts or plastic flap. Primary repair of nerves and tendons is not advisable.

3 *Indeterminable injuries* — these are severe crush or burn injuries where it is impossible to make early decisions about the full extent of injury. Up to 3 weeks must elapse to see what remains viable before proceeding with excision of dead tissue and repair.

The priority of treatment is repair of skin followed sequentially by management of bone and joint injury, repair of nerves and, lastly, tendon repair. Irritant solutions such as iodine and spirit should be avoided; only bland substances such as Cetrimide should be used for cleaning. Use of general anaesthetic or brachial plexus block with sedation are usually required. Careful wound toilet is performed, but live skin around the wound must be preserved. Usually the wound must be enlarged for adequate exposure, but enlarging incisions must not cross a skin crease or an interdigital web. All debris and dead tissue is excised. Fractures are reduced and, if unstable, fixation is sometimes employed. This is not devoid of risk, but stiffness in the hand from prolonged external splinting is so disabling that this is preferable. Digital nerves are best primarily repaired if skin closure is anticipated, since they may be impossible to find subsequently. Joint capsules and ligaments are sutured to restore stability and permit early movement.

Skin closure. When the tourniquet is released, meticulous haemostasis is obtained. Primary closure is performed unless the hand has been grossly contaminated. Direct suture is preferred, if this can be achieved without tension and with only slight undercutting of the skin edges. Split skin grafts are used to cover defects on the back of the hand. They are taken from the forearm and sutured into place. On the palm, a split thickness graft will contract and full thickness grafts are required. This graft is more difficult in that its vascularity is more precarious. Adequate fixation and mobilisation is therefore important. Free skin grafts will not take on a base of bone, cartilage or tendon. Flap grafts with a vascular pedicle are then required and are taken from local or distant sites. Thenar, palmar or cross finger flaps are useful for amputated finger tips. Distant pedicle flaps are reserved for severe injuries. The donor site may be the abdomen, chest or arm. Sometimes a severely mutilated finger is sacrificed and its skin used as a rotation flap. The repair is covered with a thin layer of paraffin gauze, several thicknesses of dry gauze and wool soaked in a fixative-

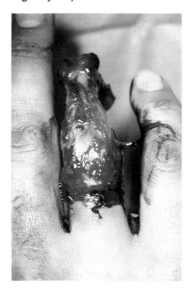

Fig 11.5 Avulsion injury of ring finger requiring amputation. The ring had become entangled in moving machinery.

paraffin emulsion. A firm crepe bandage ensures even pressure and a light plaster slab holds the wrist and hand with metacarpo phalageal joints in flexion.

The timing of tendon repair is well defined. Tidy injuries are dealt with immediately. In untidy and inderterminable injuries, repair is delayed until the wounds have healed. Amputation of a finger as a primary procedure should be avoided unless the damage involves many tissues and is clearly irreparable (Fig 11.5). Even when a finger is amputated by injury, the possibility of reattachment should be considered.

Torso wounds

Wounds of the torso are not as common as wounds elsewhere on the body, despite the high number of other types of injuries to this area. Those wounds that are seen are potentially very serious because of possible damage to the underlying vital organs. Penetrating injuries such as stab and gunshot wounds are of particular concern. Large wounds may occur as a result of road accidents where objects on or in the vehicle may penetrate the torso. Here, the wound is of secondary importance to the overall condition of the patient as other life-saving procedures may be necessary before the actual wound is considered. When it is, however, it should be carefully cleaned under strict aseptic conditions and the area may be enlarged to allow proper examination to exclude injury to the underlying organs and removal of foreign bodies.

Burns and scalds, particularly those from hot liquids, occur frequently in children who reach up to high cooker surfaces and pull over saucepans containing milk or water. Many of these scalds are quite extensive requiring admission to hospital for generalised and specific treatment including skin grafting.

Finally, wounds to the genitalia are not uncommon. Causes include lacerations from falling astride objects such as fences and in particular the cross-bar and seats of bicycles. Contusions and lacerations to the penis from being caught in a fly zip and other self-inflicted injuries also occur from time to time. Some of these injuries may be serious and internal damage such as rupture of the urethra must be excluded by careful examination of the wounds and an accurate history of how the wound was caused.

Lower limb wounds

Feet and toes tend to take the brunt of injuries to the lower limbs. The commonest are heavy objects dropped onto toes, stubbing of toes and treading on sharp objects while not wearing shoes or, at best, inadequate foot wear. Many of these are minor wounds which require only cleaning and dressing, but some may involve extensive soft tissue and bony damage. Among these are the accidents which occur with lawn mowers when toes have been severely damaged or traumatically amputated.

Dogs take a particular liking to legs and dog bites are a common occurrence. The same treatment applies as for dog bites on any other part of the anatomy, with careful wound toilet and suturing if necessary.

Grazing to the knees occurs after falls, especially in children. These wounds may be deep and full of dirt and grit and cleaning of the area must be thorough if the wound is to heal well. They are also very painful but, provided they are relatively clean, rapid regeneration of epithelium can occur if a suitable occlusive dressing is applied.

Wounds to the legs resulting from road accidents may be very severe as in compound factures of the tibia and fibula. These fractures and wounds should always be treated in an

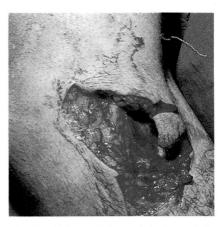

Fig 11.6 Deep laceration to right knee following a motorcycle accident.

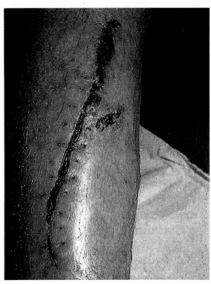

Fig 11.7 Shin laceration after removal of sutures showing residual inflammation.

operating theatre under strict aseptic conditions and the patients should be given prophylactic antibiotics since the risk of osteomyelitis is high (Fig 11.6).

One of the most problematic injuries of the lower limbs is that of deep laceration over the shin. This is especially so in the elderly whose skin is often papery thin and slow to heal. Necrosis of the skin in this area is common and healing by granulation may take many weeks. Some, however, heal more successfully as illustrated in Fig 11.7.

Wounds of the lower limb can be very incapacitating causing enforced immobilisation and time off work. Patients should be treated sympathetically and given adequate advice to enable them to cope with their situation and return to a normal lifestyle as soon as possible.

CASE STUDY 1

Mrs S, a 56-year-old lady, was a back seat passenger in a car involved in a head on collision. She was knocked unconcious, but on arrival at the A & E department was fully conscious but drowsy. On examination her

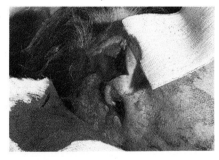

(a)

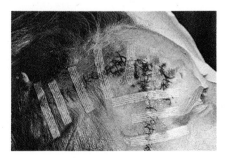

(b)

Fig 11.8 (a) Flap laceration of right temple. (b) Laceration following suture and tape closure.

injuries were found to be extensive bruising to both legs, right shoulder and face, a large laceration of her right shin and a severe 'flap' laceration to her right temple (Fig 11.8a). Neurological examination and observations showed no deficit. Intramuscular ampicillin and flucloxacillin (Magnapen®) was given and a tetanus toxoid course started. Under general anaesthesia her wounds were sutured and tape-closed (Fig 11.8b). Approximation of the skin edges was good and there was no skin loss.

Mrs S made an uneventful recovery and was discharged 4 days after her accident. Her sutures were removed on a return visit to the A & E department and both wounds had healed well.

CASE STUDY 2

Mr N, a 39-year-old self-employed coppice worker, struck his left thumb with an axe while chopping wood. He arrived in the A & E

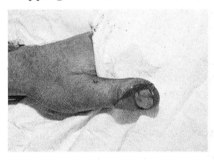

Fig 11.9 Laceration of left thumb.

department with a deep laceration running obliquely across the top of his thumb (Fig 11.9). An x-ray revealed an oblique fracture of the distal phalynx. Under a ring block anaesthetic the wound was thoroughly cleaned and sutured.

The wound was redressed at regular intervals to observe any signs of infection. The sutures were removed after 8 days when the wound had healed without any problems. Gradual mobilisation of the thumb was encouraged and the patient was discharged after 3 weeks.

CASE STUDY 3

Mr L, a 40-year-old building contractor, caught his right heel on a paving slab while working on a building site sustaining a large laceration over the Achilles tendon (Fig 11.10). The tendon, though exposed, was fortunately intact, requiring wound toilet and suturing of the skin. A firm supportive bandage was applied and Mr L was advised to rest his leg as much as possible. The wound was redressed 3 days later when it was found to be inflamed, tender and the whole foot very swollen. A course of ampicillin capsules was started and Mr L was advised to rest his leg completely, but to do gentle, active movements of his toes and ankle. At his next visit the swelling and inflammation had subsided

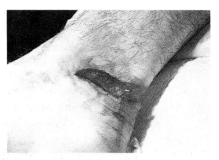

Fig 11.10   Laceration of ankle over Achilles tendon.

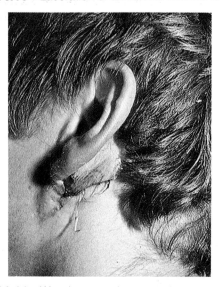

Fig 11.11   Wood penetrating posterior auricular region.

and subsequently the wound healed well. The sutures were removed after 10 days.

CASE STUDY 4

Mr C, an 18-year-old, fell against a tree while 'messing about' with his friends and a 5 cm wedge of wood pierced the skin in the left posterior auricular region burrowing under the skin to reach the angle of his jaw. He arrived in the A & E department with the piece of wood *in situ* (Fig 11.11). A local anaesthetic was administered and the piece of wood was removed. The wound was further examined and cleaned and skin sutures applied to the puncture wound. A tetanus toxoid injection was given and Mr C returned 1 week later when the sutures were removed to reveal a neat, well healed scar.

CRITICAL ASSESSMENT OF CASE STUDIES

The patients presented have a typical collection of minor wounds seen from day-to-day in any accident department. In each case the outcome was satisfactory, but the treatment less than ideal for the following reasons:

Case 1

This lady was given an unnecessary general anaesthetic soon after a period of unconsciousness and whilst in a postconcussional state. Though neurological examination was said to be unremarkable, the blow to the right temple was clearly severe in order to produce a laceration of the magnitude shown (Fig 11.8a). A combination of a non psychotropic analgesic (Codeine phosphate) together with local anaesthetic could have been used so as to be able to monitor her neurological state continuously and rule out an extradural haematoma. Alternatively, dressings could have been applied to the wounds with suture at a later stage. There is no real indication for antibiotics since the wounds were not heavily contaminated and there were no associated fractures. Wound toilet is all that was required apart from tetanus prophylaxis if not up to date. Silk sutures are less than ideal for facial wounds, fine nylon is more appropriate. Alternatively, the underlying fascial layers could have been accurately approximated with absorbable sutures and the skin with tapes. Combinations of sutures and tapes are rarely necessary.

Case 2

This is a contaminated traumatic laceration with compound fracture even if the bone was not visible at the laceration site (Fig 11.9). It is extremely difficult to clean such a wound adequately and therefore it should not have been sutured primarily. There is a case for antibiotics in the presence of open bony injury. An occlusive dressing and early mobilisation would have provided an equally good result without the risk of infection in a primarily closed contaminated wound.

Case 3

Another contaminated wound closed primarily and this time resulting in wound infection (Fig 11.10). Blind broad spectrum antibiotic treatment was given, fortunately with success. In the presence of established infection, removal of sutures with local wound drainage and culture of exudate is required. Antibiotics are best given according to the results of Gram stain or culture. Rest and evaluation of the leg are mandatory. Swelling in closed fascial compartments may lead to compromise of arterial blood supply and deep vein thrombosis. In the preantibiotic era suture of such a laceration might have led to gangrene.

Case 4

Wood splinters are usually heavily contaminated with bacteria including *Cl. tetani* or *Cl. welchii*. This was a deeply penetrating wound which should have been lightly dressed and left to heal by secondary intention (Fig 11.11). Closing the wound encourages the growth of anaerobic bacteria in the damaged tissues, and without surgical debridement, wound toilet cannot be expected to clean such wounds reliably.

In each case treatment was given with good intention, but without resort to the basic principles of wound care. The results were satisfactory, but could have been otherwise had the contaminating organisms been more virulent or unresponsive to the antibiotics given. Every traumatic wound is an exercise in bacteriology. Apposition of the wound edges may be reassuring for the patient but safety is the first consideration.

Chapter 12

Wounds caused by the Weapons of War

Michael Owen-Smith

War wounds occur not only in times of war but whenever and wherever the weapons of war are used. These weapons differ from the usual peacetime, hand-held, blunt and sharp instruments and low velocity handguns in that they produce almost exclusively high velocity fragment or bullet wounds, or explosive blast injuries.

When wounds are inflicted by low velocity handgun bullets, knives or other penetrating weapons, they can usually be managed by conventional surgical methods without too much harm. If these same procedures are used in high velocity wounds from rifle bullets or explosive blast fragments the results can be disastrous.

Surgeons and their patients have had to learn the hard way that these injuries require a different form of treatment. The correct treatment has been known since World War I and the principles have not changed much since World War II about 40 years ago. Regrettably, at the beginning of every minor or major war, there is still widespread ignorance about these methods.

MECHANISM OF INJURY

Bullet wounds

When a bullet strikes the body, the damage inflicted depends on the size, shape, stability and, above all, the velocity of the missile, and the structures with which it comes into con- tact. Bullets are divided into two groups, low velocity fired from handguns and high velocity from rifles (Fig 12.1). Handguns may be revolvers or they may be automatic, but they all fire a fairly heavy bullet at relatively low velocities of 200–300 metres per second (700–1000 feet per second). A typical military or hunting rifle fires a bullet of about 10 g at over 800 mps (2600 fps). Rifles of this type have been in existence for over 100 years. Present and future developments in military rifles are towards smaller bullets fired at an even higher velocity. For example, the Colt Armalite rifle of calibre 5.56 mm fires a very small bullet weighing 3.5 g at a velocity of about 1000 mps (3250 fps) and the Russian AK74, now in use in Afghanistan, is similar. Pistol bullets have a relatively low amount of energy available to cause damage and in general this only occurs at fairly close range (below 100 metres). They simply core out a hole through the body and, like a knife, only damage those tissues which they actually touch; there is no hidden damage. On the other hand, all rifle bullets have an incredible amount of energy to cause severe wounding even at ranges of 500–1000 metres. They transfer this energy by the process of 'cavitation' and shock waves. These happen so quickly that ultra high speed cinephotography is required to record it.

Temporary cavitation only occurs with high velocity bullets and fragments and is the main reason for their immensely destructive effect.

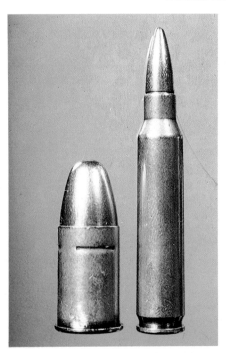

Fig 12.1 Low velocity handgun bullet (*left*); high velocity rifle bullet (*right*).

As the rifle bullet releases its energy, it is absorbed by the local tissues which are violently accelerated forwards and outwards. A large cavity is, therefore, created which is approximately 30–40 times the diameter of the missile. The maximum size of the cavity is reached only after the bullet has passed through the tissues. It has a subatmospheric pressure and is open at both entrance and exit holes. The temporary cavity collapses in a pulsatile fashion rather like a concertina, sucking air, debris and surface bacteria into the wound. All these wounds are grossly contaminated and there is a large amount of dead tissue. Some tissues are much more sensitive to the cavitational changes than others.

In general, the damage is ¡directly proportional to the density of the tissue and, therefore, homogenous tissues like muscle, liver, spleen and brain are very sensitive, whereas the light tissues such as the lung, which is mainly filled with air, are resistant. The damage is also inversely proportional to the amount of elastic fibres present; for example,

skin and lung are remarkably resistant to such damage whereas bone is very sensitive.

The external appearance of a bullet wound can be deceptive because the skin is so elastic that there may well be tiny entrance and exit holes which hide extremely severe wounds. In a rifle bullet wound a volume of tissue may be destroyed which is equal to the size of a fist. This large amount of dead tissue, uniformly and grossly contaminated with bacteria, clostridial spores, clothing and debris from the surface is the pathological entity of the high velocity missle wound and does not occur with any other wound.

In wounds containing dead tissue, particularly muscle, the conditions are right for the development of clostridial myonecrosis or gas gangrene. It must be remembered that this is a clinical diagnosis not a bacteriological one and it is the one condition which, above all other infections, must be prevented. It was the main reason why the principles of thorough wound excision and delayed primary wound closure were developed and made mandatory in war surgery. This mandatory treatment must be extended to include all high velocity missile wounds whenever and wherever they occur.

Explosive blast injuries

Explosives are substances which, when detonated, are changed almost instantaneously from solid or liquid form into a vast volume of gases. The body can be damaged by three separate physical phenomena associated with an explosive blast. These are fragments from the bomb, blast pressure waves and blast wind.

The fragments which come off an explosive device travel at high velocity. They are not streamlined like bullets and, therefore, at a distance from the explosion they become low velocity missiles. In wartime, more than 80% of all injuries are caused by fragments from explosive devices and, similarly, homemade bombs which are packed with nails, screws, ballbearings and other debris can create a large number of injuries (Fig 12.2).

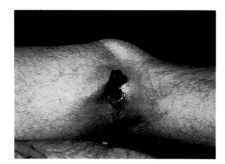

Fig 12.2 Knee injury caused by a 6in bolt from a homemade bomb.

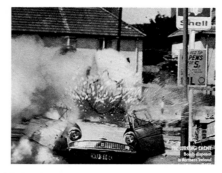

Fig 12.3 A car bomb explosion. (By courtesy of *The Sunday Telegraph*.)

The blast pressure wave is created by explosive gases compressing the surrounding air. This zone of compression moves away from the site of the explosion at high speed as a sphere of rapidly increasing radius. Although the pressure wave does not last for long, it can reach very high pressures of thousands of pounds per square inch. Like sound waves, pressure waves will flow over and around an obstruction so that someone hiding behind a wall may be affected by a pure pressure wave. These waves are similar to radio waves in that they will pass right through the body and it is only those parts which contain air or gas which are damaged. The ears, the lungs and the gas-containing viscera are the most vulnerable areas.

The blast wind, or mass movement of air, is caused by the displacement of air by the vast volume of explosive gas. This rushes away from the explosion at high speed in excess of the speed of Concorde in flight (Fig 12.3). According to the velocity of the wind the body may simply be blown over, thrown many metres or thrown against the surrounding environment causing acceleration and deceleration injuries.

Closer to the explosion, the blast wind may simply blow pieces off the body — all variations occur in proportion to the violence of the explosion and the velocity of the blast wind. In a massive explosion, the body may be totally disintegrated and atomised. Lower levels may cause total disruption of the body or it may be blown into a few or more pieces. Lesser levels will cause traumatic amputation varying from the whole of the limb to parts of the limb or digit (Fig 12.4). These traumatic amputations are quite common after explosions. When they occur in confined spaces, up to a quarter of all the dead and seriously injured victims may have traumatic amputations.

PRINCIPLES OF SURGERY OF WAR WOUNDS

A high velocity bullet or fragment wound causes a large amount of dead and pulped muscle, grossly contaminated with bacteria, debris, clothing and dirt sucked in from the outside environment. The majority of such wounds are of soft tissue and the remainder involve special tissues such as bone, blood vessels, brain or the internal organs of the trunk.

Wounds of soft tissue

The treatment of a soft tissue wound is a two-stage procedure, the first operation is wound excision which is followed at an interval of 4–5 days by delayed primary closure of the wound. In peacetime, these operations may be done in one hospital and under the supervision of the same surgeon, whereas in wartime it is usual for the two operations to be done by different surgeons at different hospitals on the route of evacuation of the casualty

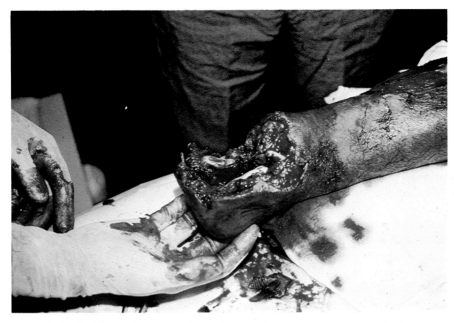

Fig 12.4 Traumatic amputation of the foot from an antipersonnel mine.

from the point of wounding back to base hospitals. It is important, therefore, that the records include a good description of the parts that have been wounded and any damage to important structures, the type of weapon causing the wound and the method of treatment, including a simple diagram of the wound both in the record and on any plaster cast that may have been used.

Wound excision

Wound excision is the process whereby grossly contaminated, dead and damaged tissue is thoroughly excised (sometimes called debridement). This leaves an area of healthy tissue with a good blood supply, capable of combating residual infection provided that the wound is not primarily closed. The technique of wound excision is as follows: the clothing, dressings and splints are carefully removed and a sterile gauze pad is held over the wound, whilst the surrounding area of skin and the whole circumference of the limb, when involved, is cleansed with detergent, shaved, dried and then painted with an antiseptic. In the case of multiple wounds, the posterior aspect of body and limb should be dealt with

before those on the anterior aspect in order to minimise the stress of turning the patient (Fig 12.5).

The skin is very resistant to damage; only pulped or dead skin should be excised and this means that no more than 2 mm of skin from the edges of the wound should ever be re-

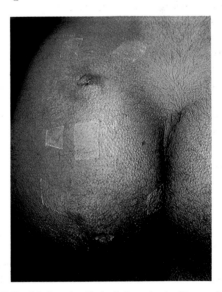

Fig 12.5 High velocity bullet wound with small entry and exit holes.

moved. In order to get to the depths of the wound, the skin should be incised generously; in the limbs the incision should be in the long axis, but not over subcutaneous bone or across flexion creases. The subcutaneous fat and the shredded superficial fascia about the wound are always contaminated and should be thoroughly excised.

The deep fascia must be incised along the length of the incision. This essential step allows wide and deep retraction without tension and thus enables the depths of the wound to be exposed. It may be necessary to add transverse cuts to the deep fascia at either end of the wound in order to improve access. Undamaged fascial compartments may need decompression in order to avoid ischaemic changes due to post-traumatic oedema.

The edges of the wound should be retracted and blood clots, dirt, debris and missiles removed from the sides and the depths of the wound. Gentle but copious irrigation with saline or water will wash out most residual debris and blood clots. The wound should be explored with the finger to identify foreign bodies and unexpected extensions of the wound, but fresh planes in healthy tissue should not be opened up. Clinical and radiological localisation may indicate that the foreign bodies can be approached by separate incisions through fascial planes rather than by cutting through healthy muscle. Excision of dead muscle must be thorough as dead muscle is the ideal medium for Clostridial sepsis leading to gas gangrene. The permanent track of the missile is the one you can see, but this track is surrounded by dead muscle and it is this which must always be excised. All muscle which is not healthy and red, which does not contract when pinched with forceps or bleed when cut, *must* be excised until healthy, contractile, bleeding muscle is reached. The technique for this is to use scissors and to excise small lumps of dead muscle but always taking into account the anatomy of the region and the vital structures which must be preserved if they are not grossly damaged. Haemostasis should be by pressure with warm packs and the use of ligatures of fine non-absorbable material or Dexon to bleeding points. These must be picked up accurately in order to leave as little dead tissue as is possible. For the same reason diathermy coagulation should not be used as it is important not to leave any dead tissue behind for residual Clostridia to multiply in. The widely opened deep fascia is left open to allow postoperative oedematous and congested tissue to swell without tension, thus avoiding interference with the blood supply (Fig 12.6).

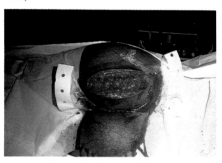

Fig 12.6 Wide excision of dead muscle from wound.

Limitation of closure

All wounds should be left open without suture of the skin or deep structures with the following exceptions:

Face and neck. These wounds may be closed primarily after wound excision.

Head injuries. The dura must be closed, by suture or by temporalis fascia graft, and the skin closed by rotating flaps to provide cover.

Soft tissues of the chest wall. The wound must be excised and healthy muscle must be closed over sucking chest wounds in order to establish an airtight closure, but the skin should be left open.

Soft tissues of the abdominal wall. The wound must be excised and the peritoneum closed together with a layer of healthy muscle to allow a watertight closure, but the superficial layers and the skin must be left open.

Joints. The synovial membrane must be

closed; if this is not possible, then the capsule alone should be closed. If the capsule cannot be closed, the joint is left open and immobilised in the position of function.

Hand injuries. Some injuries may be closed primarily, but usually they are left open for delayed primary closure. Tendon and nerve should be covered and all viable tissue should be preserved as this simplifies reconstructive procedures.

Blood vessels. Those vessels that have been repaired should be covered by healthy muscle.

Dressings

Dry gauze is laid across the open wound and this is covered by a bulky, fluffed up, absorbent dressing (Fig 12.7). Tulle gras should not be used and the wound should not be packed in any way with the dressing as this will form a plug and prevent an easy outflow of the bacterial-laden inflammatory exudate from the wound. The whole dressing should be held in place by some form of sticky plaster applied longitudinally, for the strapping must never be placed right round the limb. In all cases where there is an extensive soft tissue wound, the limb as a whole should be immobilised; this is best done with splints, well padded plasters which *must* be split down to the skin at the time the plaster is applied, or best of all, plaster of Paris slabs.

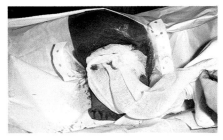

Fig 12.7 Dry dressing applied to wound covered with fluffed up gauze.

Delayed primary closure

Provided that the wound resulting from a high velocity missile injury has been thoroughly excised, there should be no necessity for further inspection of the wound until the time comes for closure. When there is a specific indication such as excessive pain, oedema or signs of infection, it will be necessary to inspect the wound in the operating theatre under a general anaesthetic. This usually means that wound excision was incomplete and further excision of dead tissue is necessary. This mistake should be avoided if at all possible and thorough excision usually comes with experience of the technique, but with good training a surgeon's first attempt at excision should be successful.

When initial wound excision has been adequate, the open missile wound will continue to ooze blood and serum for 2 days. The wound is sealed with coagulated serum by the 3rd day and early granulations appear over the surface of the fibrinous coagulum between the 3rd and 5th days. This period forms the best time for delayed closure of such wounds. Closure earlier than the 3rd day or later than the 5th day results in a higher failure rate of primary healing. At first this time was found empirically, but has now been proven experimentally by controlled trials.

At operation, the wound is disturbed as little as possible; the edges are separated and any blood clot which is present is carefully removed by gentle and copious irrigation with saline or water. Inevitably, these excised missile wounds tend to gape, but this should not cause undue alarm provided that there has been no significant loss of skin. The wound should be thoroughly inspected and any tiny tags of dead tissue which have been missed should be excised. In deeper wounds the track should be explored in case anything has been missed in the primary operation (Fig 12.8). No deep sutures are inserted and drainage is avoided wherever possible. The skin edges may be undermined if necessary in order to provide cover without tension on the sutured edges. Such a procedure is safe in most areas up to a depth of 8 cm. Great care must be taken over haemostasis, the dead space must

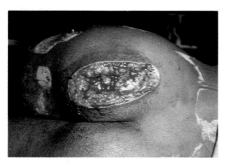

Fig 12.8 Wound after removal of dressing showing only slight surface contamination.

be obliterated and the finished suture line must not be under any tension. Only fine suture material should be used for the skin because, if there is any tension, it means that there is a chance that the wound will break down. Any remaining area is covered by split skin grafts. The sutured, or grafted, wound is then dressed and, if it is on a limb, it should be placed at rest in a padded plaster splint. The wound does not need to be disturbed for 7–10 days unless there is a specific indication. If there is an indication that all is not going well, the wound should be inspected in theatre. Extensive wounds can only be closed satisfactorily by plastic methods and elaborate work of this nature should be the responsibility of the plastic surgeon.

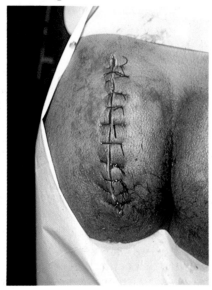

Fig 12.9 Delayed primary closure of the wound.

About 95% of missile wounds are suitable for delayed primary closure and uncomplicated healing occurs in well over 90% (Fig 12.9).

The infected wound

This is usually due to inadequate primary wound excision. Such a wound will need a second operation to ensure that all dead tissue is excised, the appropriate antibiotic will have to be used and thorough drainage ensured. If it is only minor sepsis that responds rapidly to treatment, the wound may still be closed by delayed primary suture; but major sepsis will mean that the wound cannot be closed in this way and will need closure by secondary suture or graft once the infection is completely under control.

When circumstances are poor, there may be occasions when a large number of untreated wounds may be admitted long after the infliction of the wound. After a time lag of more than 12 hours, major surgical interference is likely to do more harm than good and will spread sepsis. In such cases, removal of dead tissue, relief of tension, evacuation of haematomata and adequate drainage is the only surgery that is advisable. This must be accomplished by incising the wound widely, removing all necrotic tissues and accessible foreign bodies and commencing appropriate antibiotic therapy.

The aim in surgery of all missile wounds is to treat such wounds within 6 hours; it is important to remember this time interval from wounding to surgery when planning surgical cover for a number of patients who have been injured by missiles.

Wounds of bones and joints

Between 60 and 75% of all missile wounds and blast injuries involve the upper and lower extremities and, therefore, such a wound is usually the first type of missile wound a surgeon is called upon to treat (Fig 12.10). The management of a compound fracture is very similar to that of a soft tissue wound

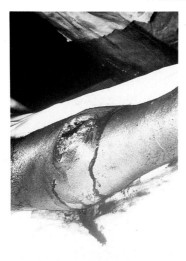

Fig 12.10   Rifle bullet wound of leg.

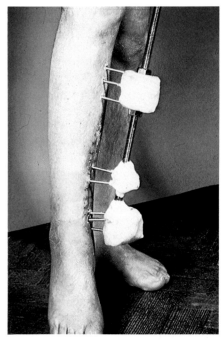

Fig 12.11   External fixation device to immobilise a compound fracture from a shell fragment wound.

already described, but with the special addition of injury to bone and any associated injuries to blood vessels and nerves.

Bone is commonly shattered into a number of pieces; tiny fragments without any attachments should be discarded, but all other fragments with periosteum or muscle attachment should be cleaned thoroughly using a sharp curette and copious irrigation and replaced.

Any large attached fragment, particularly if it contributes to maintaining the length of the bone, should be cleaned and replaced and the major bone ends brought roughly into line. The soft tissues are excised as has been described; repair of the major blood vessels to the limb must be performed at the earliest stage of the operation, as failure to do this jeopardises the survival of the limb. Severed nerves are marked and their positions noted, damaged tendons are trimmed, but no attempt should be made at primary repair in either case.

Internal fixation of bones should not be done in these injuries, even when required to protect an accompanying arterial anastomosis, because of the gross and unacceptable risk of sepsis. However, external fixation using pins placed through normal tissues above and

below the fractures is permitted and thoroughly recommended (Fig 12.11). After delayed primary closure and when primary wound healing has taken place, further procedures on the bone, nerves or tendons can be done at leisure.

Vascular injuries

Injuries to major blood vessels require prompt surgical treatment if the tissues supplied by these vessels are to be salvaged. Most acute vascular injuries which require surgical repair involve peripheral vessels. Very few patients with injuries of major vessels of abdominal or thoracic cavities ever survive to reach hospital.

Time is at a premium in vascular injuries, the vessels should be repaired and the blood supply to the peripheral tissues restored as soon as possible, in any case within 6 hours. At operation, wound excision has to follow control of haemorrhage. The damaged ends are trimmed until macroscopically normal vessel is reached and 20 to 40 ml of heparinised saline is injected distally. If free back bleeding is not obtained, a size 3 or 4 Fogarty balloon catheter should be passed and withdrawn before injecting heparinised saline. The deep veins are as important to repair as arteries and similar methods should be used. A simple laceration of a vessel caused by a low velocity missile can be repaired by lateral suture. A vessel that has been severed, or has a segment destroyed by a high velocity missile, must be repaired using autogenous vein graft. Synthetic prosthesis must not be used due to the grave and unacceptable risk of infection. Usually a reversed saphenous graft is used and anastomoses are made obliquely, in order to gain maximum diameter using 5.0 or 6.0 atraumatic sutures. After repair and completion of wound excision, the vessels are covered by healthy muscle, fasciotomy is usually performed, and the wound left open for delayed primary closure.

Chest wounds

Direct damage to the chest from penetrating wounds may involve the chest wall, lungs, mediastinal contents, heart and diaphragm. The lung itself is remarkably resistant whereas the heart and mediastinal contents are extremely susceptible to cavitation damage.

It is essential that pleural and pericardial spaces be kept empty and that their normal pressures be maintained. This requires release of tension pneumothorax, aspiration of the pericardium for cardiac tamponade, the closure of an open penumothorax, stabilisation of a stove-in chest and drainage of a large pneumothorax or haemothorax. Bleeding from penetrating chest wounds is usually from intercostal or internal mammary vessels; the lung itself does not usually bleed much and massive haemorrhage from major pulmonary vessels is rapidly fatal. The basis of treatment is withdrawal of the blood-stained effusion from the pleural space and replacement of the measured blood loss. If clinical examination reveals signs of blood or air in the pleural space, a wide-bore intercostal drainage tube should be inserted through the lateral chest wall in the mid-

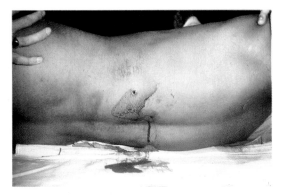

Fig 12.12 Tiny entrance wound in the chest from a 7.62 mm rifle bullet. The exit wound was equally small.

axillary line for removal of blood and fluid. This should be attached to a Heimlich one-way valve and thence in a closed system to a drainage bag. Underwater seal suction drainage should be applied as soon as is practicable. A chest x-ray should be taken afterwards to confirm the location of the tube and evacuation of the pleural space, and to locate any foreign bodies. The tube may be removed when there is no longer any evidence of air leak, when the lung is fully expanded and when air and fluid are no longer present in the pleural cavity. An accurate record should be made of the amount of blood loss through the chest drain.

War experience has shown that over 85% of all penetrating and perforating wounds of the chest may be managed by closed-tube thoracostomy (Fig 12.12). Thoracotomy is required for specific indications such as continued intrathoracic bleeding, massive and continuing air leakage, abdominothoracic injury, injury to the mediastinal contents, cardiac wounds, sucking wounds of the chest and large wounds of the chest wall where there is a defect. When thoracotomy is required, most chest wounds may be dealt with through the standard posterolateral thoracotomy. Bleeding from the lung usually ends once the lung has been inflated and comes into contact with the chest wall, but in some lung wounds ligation of bleeding vessels and oversewing of a small segment of the lung may be necessary; pulmonary resection is seldom required.

Abdominal wounds

Penetrating missile wounds of the abdomen require urgent treatment because a patient who has been wounded in the abdomen is almost certain to die unless he is operated upon. Small calibre bullets and high velocity fragments from explosive devices may produce minute superficial wounds which can be associated with amazingly severe internal damage (Fig 12.13). Early operation is mandatory as part of the resuscitation process, the commonest cause of death is haemorrhage and this requires treatment at the earliest possible moment, whereas the closure of intestinal leaks is less urgent. After passing a catheter into the bladder a full laparotomy incision should be made; for severe injuries a generous full length mid-line incision is quickest and best. Haemorrhage is dealt with first, followed by repair of all perforations of the alimentary tract.

Perforations of the small bowel and the stomach may be closed by suture in the usual fashion. Resection of small gut should be performed when the group of perforations is so close that their repair would overlap or when the injury is on the mesenteric border; end-to-end anastomosis should be done by the surgeon's usual technique and the result should be good.

Wounds of the colon occur almost as frequently as those of the small intestine. They are usually more serious because the blood supply is not so good and the contents of the large bowel escape more readily and are highly infective. Perforations of the colon should be looked for most carefully because those in the fixed portions and on the mesenteric aspects of the transverse colon are difficult to demonstrate and are easily missed. The colon must be mobilised in order to get a good view of it; any part of the wall of the colon which is contused or discoloured should be repaired, resected or exteriorised. There are three basic methods of treating colon injuries by missiles:

1 Exteriorisation of the damaged or repaired colon.
2 Repair by suture, with or without proximal colostomy.
3 Resection with or without primary anastomosis.

Due to difficulties with its liquid contents, the right colon should *not* be exteriorised, but the transverse and descending colon are readily exteriorised and this method is still very useful on occasions, particularly under field conditions or when postoperative care is minimal. The method of treatment used will depend on the severity of damage to the colon. Major disrupted segmental damage caused by a high velocity wound should be treated by resection and the formation of a colostomy, or ileostomy, and a distal mucous fistula (Fig 12.14). Moderate wounds may be treated by resection, anastomosis and proximal defunctioning colostomy. A damaged segment of transverse or left colon may be mobilised and exteriorised as a large loop colostomy. Finally, simple repair of a perforation should be reserved for the uncomplicated, low velocity wound with minimal damage to the colon and no complicating factors.

A thorough peritoneal toilet and lavage with warm saline or an antibiotic solution such as 1 g tetracycline per litre should be followed by thorough dependent drainage and closure of the laparotomy wound with retention sutures. Good pelvic drainage can be achieved by excision of the tip of the coccyx, placing drains well

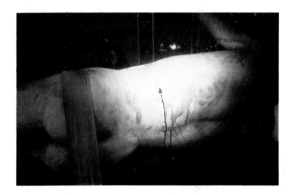

Fig 12.13 Exit wound of an Armalite rifle bullet wound of the abdomen.

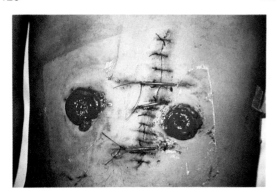

Fig 12.14 Resection of disrupted transverse colon from a major HVM wound, formation of colostomy and mucous fistula. (By courtesy of Mr Adrian Boyd.)

up into the space between the sacrum and rectum.

Wounds of the rectum should be treated by repair or resection and anastomosis, thorough drainage and the formation of an efficient defunctioning colostomy. The distal rectal segment should be irrigated and thoroughly cleansed at the time of initial surgery and adequate drainage of the retrorectal space provided.

Liver injuries should be treated by excision of the damaged tissue, haemostasis and very thorough drainage. Wounds of the spleen are treated by splenectomy. Pancreatic injuries require repair and thorough drainage if minor or involving the head of the pancreas, whereas severe injuries of the body of the tail may require resection and drainage.

MORTALITY

The mortality from missile wounds and explosive blast injury is high. Even when the best facilities are available, together with a short evacuation time, the mortality is about 18%. If relatively minor injuries are excluded, the mortality rises to between 20 and 25% and if high velocity penetrating or perforating missile injuries alone are included the mortality rate exceeds 30%. Mortality is 4–5 times higher for high velocity wounds than for low velocity bullet and stab wounds.

The important factors that influence mortality and morbidity rates are:

The type of missile — with a high or low velocity.
The part of the body that is hit.
The organs that are damaged.
The delay before surgery.

All these variables must be clearly separated and defined before any comparison of various series of gunshot wounds is made.

The principles of management of high velocity missile wounds are based upon millions of patients and many thousands of surgeons' experience. These principles and simple methods work. They have stood the test of time and many patients have had to suffer in the past when surgeons have had to relearn these principles the hard way in every war or every situation that involves high velocity missile wounds.

Chapter 13

The Management of Compound Fractures

Michael Beverly and Richard Coombs

Compound or open fractures typically affect the young and active. Careful management restores normal function and a full life while inadequate treatment leads to chronic osteomyelitis, disuse osteoporosis and potential amputation. Open fractures, previously associated with battle and violent sport, are now more frequently seen following road traffic accidents, particularly those involving the unprotected pedestrian or motor-cyclist (Fig 13.1).

Just as the common aetiology has changed so has orthodox management. Cautery, crude splintage and amputation have given way to routine antibiotics, reliable fixation and early mobilisation.

PRINCIPLES OF MANAGEMENT

Experience gained in war has served to emphasise certain important principles in the management of open fractures. Such injuries are surgical emergencies. They require early and thorough exploration. All foreign material and dead tissue must be carefully removed in one or more procedures. All contaminated wounds or those associated with any tissue of doubtful viability must be left open.

The optimum timing for skin closure will vary and must be selected with care. Clean wounds may be closed immediately, but those wounds caused by high velocity projectiles or crushing injuries, often contaminated with clo-

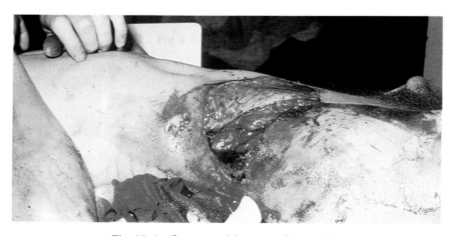

Fig 13.1 Compound fracture of the pelvis.

thing, road dirt or oil, must be left open. The availability of elegant methods for immediate fixation must not divert attention from the care of the soft tissues.

Initial assessment and treatment

Open fractures are serious injuries seldom occurring in isolation. Associated chest, abdominal and intracranial problems must be excluded. A specialised accident surgeon may assess and treat all these problems but, more usually, a number of specialists are involved and priorities must be quickly established.

Resuscitation

A clear airway and adequate circulation are crucial. An endotracheal tube and assisted ventilation may be required. Lost blood is replaced initially with saline or plasma expanders and then, as soon as possible, with cross-matched blood. Frank haemorrhage is controlled by local pressure and venous ooze is reduced by elevation of the part. After a head injury routine quarter-hourly neurological assessments are commenced.

History

Details of the accident are helpful in defining the extent and type of injury and may be obtained from witnesses or ambulance men. Was there a high or low velocity injury? Was there a sharp blow or a crushing force? Has the patient's condition been affected by drugs, alcohol or a serious medical problem? Was an epileptic fit, a heart attack, a stroke or diabetes the cause of this accident? How may these factors affect orthopaedic management?

Physical examination

A full physical examination is mandatory. Detailed assessment of the injury may have to await general anaesthesia, but the surgeon must be aware of potential occult problems. All four limbs are palpated and their movement assessed. Pulses distal to the site of the injury are sought and, where equivocal, are confirmed with a Doppler machine. Peripheral nerve function is carefully tested and recorded. The chest, heart, abdomen and neurological systems are specifically examined for signs of trauma.

Preoperative investigation

Preoperative x-rays must be taken of all potentially fractured bones and will help to exclude foreign bodies in open wounds. Head injuries are often associated with cervical spine fractures and the neck should always be x-rayed if the patient has been knocked unconscious. Similarly, femoral neck fractures are often associated with fractures of the knee or lower femoral shaft. The full length of any fractured bone must be x-rayed to exclude a double injury (Fig. 13.2).

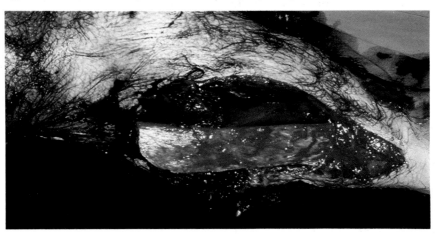

Fig 13.2 Compound fracture of the tibia.

Fluids and drugs

Several pints of blood may be lost from the circulation after a pelvic or femoral fracture and initial resuscitation must replace this as quickly as possible.

Prophylactic antibiotics are essential for all compound fractures. A broad spectrum penicillin or cephalosporin, often combined with a second antibiotic specifically active against staphylococci, is given parenterally.

A course of tetanus immunisation for unprotected individuals is mandatory with all open wounds and, together with prophylactic antibiotics, should prevent this otherwise frequently fatal complication. No wound is too trivial for these precautions: tetanus may follow a simple graze. Antitetanus serum may be used in heavily contaminated wounds, but care is required to monitor and treat any anaphylactic reaction.

Opiate analgesia is ideal for pain relief, but should be avoided in head and chest injuries. Steroids may help to minimise the effects of fat embolism, the crush syndrome and cerebral oedema. Generally, they should be used in large doses for short periods with adequate antibiotic cover. They may themselves induce serious gastrointestinal haemorrhage or psychoses.

Fat embolism

After serious injury to the long bones, fat globules may appear in the blood, urine and sputum. The total blood fat content may not be increased, but normal emulsification is altered. Fat globules may then block the arterioles in the lungs, brains, spinal cord and retina.

In the lung, fat globules are hydrolysed by lung lipoprotein lipase to glycerol and free fatty acids. The latter cause a local capillary reaction with interstitial oedema. Abnormal ventilation to perfusion ratios arise with a fall in arterial Po_2. Resulting hyperventilation leads to a parallel fall in Pco_2. Petechiae appear on the chest wall and there is often a fall in serum calcium ion levels. These symptoms merge imperceptibly with the Adult Respiratory Distress Syndrome (ARDS) and may also become manifest as a bleeding disorder related to Disseminated Intravascular Coagulation (DIC), with uniformly abnormal blood clotting tests and fibrin degradation products present in blood and urine.

The importance of considering fat embolism in the patient with serious compound fractures cannot be overemphasised. If there is any doubt about a patient's condition deteriorating within a week of major accident or surgery, the blood gases must be measured and if necessary the patient intubated and ventilated with oxygen until the crisis is over.

The crush syndrome

This is characterised by shock and oliguria. The injured muscle is tense with oedema and thus ischaemic. Large amounts of myoglobin are released into the circulation, block the renal tubules and spill over into the urine.

Any severely crushed tissue must be excised from the open wound. Urgent amputation may be life saving. Copious amounts of fluid to flush the kidneys are administered by mouth or parenterally. In severe cases haemodialysis may be required.

OPERATIVE MANAGEMENT

With initial assessment and resuscitation complete, the wounds are examined under general anaesthesia in the main operating theatre (Fig. 13.3; 13.4). A pneumatic tourniquet is used only to arrest severe arterial haemorrhage. Once this is under control the cuff should be removed. Simple elevation of the limb is usually sufficient to control venous oozing.

Preparation

The wound and surrounding skin are washed with a mild antiseptic solution copiously applied with a sterile sponge or swabs. Earth, dirt or blood may be loosened and removed with dilute hydrogen peroxide and a scrub-

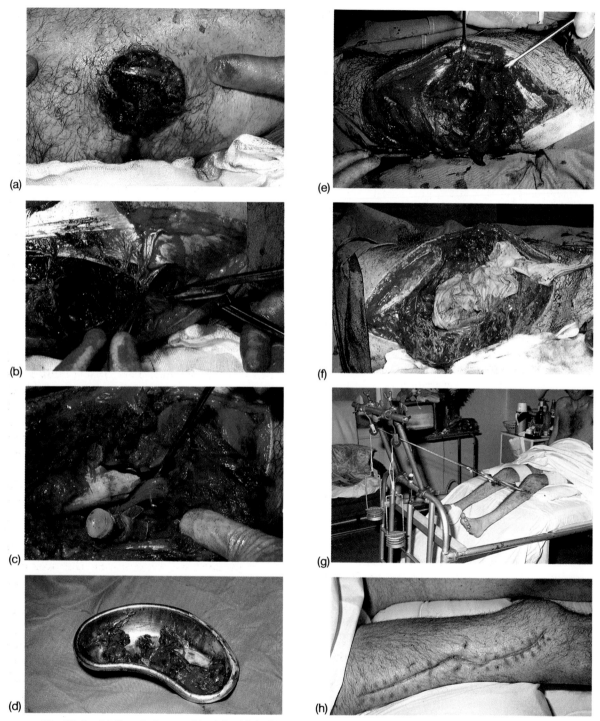

Fig 13.3 (a) Gunshot wound to right thigh; (b) Excision of debris, contaminated and devitalised tissue; (c) Cartridge case embedded in fracture site; (d) Excised material; (e) Wound debridement in an advanced stage; (f) Flavine pack inserted into cavity in thigh; (g) Skeletal traction; (h) Wound healed at 6 weeks after delayed primary closure.

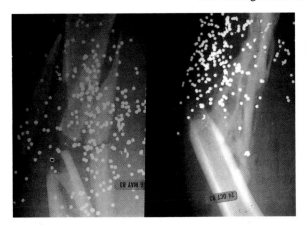

Fig 13.4 X-ray of the wound site in the patient shown in Fig 13.3.

bing brush. Multiple injuries need separate bowls and brushes to avoid cross-contamination.

The surgeon regowns and further cleans the operative area. Strong alcoholic solutions must not enter the open wound as nerves and tendons may be irreparably damaged. Mild antiseptic solutions, dilute peroxide and saline are best for the deeper parts of the wound. Aqueous povidone iodine preparations are especially useful.

Skin

Non-viable loose flaps of skin and sliced, shredded, burned or crushed edges are trimmed. Extension of the wound may be required to allow full exploration. Subcutaneous nerves, large veins and skin flexures are avoided. Allowance must be made for the possible later use of skin flaps and external fixators. Supplementary incisions to relieve tension may permit primary closure.

In the hand, wound extension by a modified Bruner incision, or a Z-plasty is advocated to avoid linear scars that lead to wound contracture and flexion deformity.

Subcutaneous fat

Loose or pedunculated fat is trimmed. To avoid devascularisation, fat and skin are mobilised together cleaving the plane below the subcutaneous fat with a finger or blunt instrument.

Deep investing fascia

Longitudinal incisions in the fascia are needed to explore torn muscles. As deep blood clot accumulates and muscle becomes oedematous, tension builds up within the enclosed fascial compartments. The vessels within the compartments become compressed and urgent decompression of each separate compartment is essential. Within a few hours muscle may become irreparably damaged and amputation inevitable. In the calf, the anterior tibial, peroneal and superficial and deep posterior compartments are often most simply decompressed by excision of a segment of fibula.

Muscle

Torn muscle retracts drawing foreign material deep into the wound. The muscle ends must be found and trimmed of dirty and dead tissue. If the transected muscles are examined in pairs, sequentially, there is less chance of missing a single retracted muscle belly. Bright red capillary bleeding generally indicates living tissue but, following a high velocity or crushing injury, it may be difficult to ascertain the point of demarcation between dead and viable tissue. The shock wave from a high velocity bullet produces a conical area of necrosis with its apex at the entry site. Full decompression will be required. Debridement must often be repeated and closure delayed for at least 2 weeks.

Pellets from shotgun injuries become buried within the muscle and it is often impossible to remove them individually. These pellets enter at relatively low velocity, cause little surrounding damage and are rapidly walled off. Clothing, wadding and pellet cases must, however, be removed diligently.

Tendon

Tendons are often transected in compound

fractures of the forearm, wrist and hand. Reflex muscle contraction draws the tendon away from the wound margin. Muscle length must be preserved or ultimate repair becomes impossible. In highly contaminated wounds, a loose approximating suture can be used. The definitive repair should be with a non-absorbable material buried within the tendon substance.

Tendon has a poor blood supply and must not be left exposed. A covering of muscle or skin preserves its viability. If possible, tendon repairs should be splinted for at least 3 weeks under minimal tension. A Kleinert technique using a rubber band and plaster to maintain flexion while permitting active extension is a very useful refinement for the management of flexor tendon injuries.

Neurovascular bundle

Preoperative assessment of the continuity of the neurovascular bundle is often difficult. The zone of anaesthesia or hypoaesthesia of the skin often appears to increase 1 to 10 days after nerve division and this may complicate the initial clinical assessment.

At operation the nerve bundles must be closely inspected and palpated and, if there is any doubt about their continuity, they must be dissected free and the epineurium incised longitudinally so that the bundles may be inspected directly, preferably with an operating microscope.

In clean lesions, where approximation without tension is possible, nerves should be trimmed and repaired immediately. Fine sutures of nylon or human hair are used. In small nerves the individual bundles are repaired separately. In larger mixed nerves careful attention to orientation is vital if any motor function is to be restored. All nerve repairs should be performed after the tourniquet has been released or an intraneural haematoma may jeopardise the result.

In heavily contaminated wounds the nerve ends are trimmed and marked with a non-absorbable suture for secondary repair as soon as infection has resolved.

With the loss of a length of nerve, mobilisation of the proximal stump may permit anastomosis without tension, but this tends to devascularise the nerve. A free nerve graft may be preferable and, in the brachial plexus for example, use of the sural nerve with the short saphenous vein or the ulna nerve with the ulna artery may allow microvascular anastomosis to the suprascapular or transverse cervical vessels giving a living graft with its own blood supply.

Arterial lesions with distal ischaemia require repair within 6 hours of injury. If there is a well established collateral circulation, complex repairs are not justified. The management of arterial injuries is considered in another chapter.

Bone

Large self-retaining retractors allow access to the fractured bone ends. Loose splinters of bone are discarded, but fragments which are still attached to muscle or periosteum are usually viable and should be retained. Occasionally, fragments of bone are collected from the roadside or elsewhere and are offered to the surgeon for replacement, but this is unwise. Sterilisation and autoclaving of bone ensures its non-viability and it may become a haven for chronic infection. Nevertheless, especially in children, a limb may be salvaged by gently washing the loose piece of bone in isotonic cleaning solution and restoring limb length with the fragment. Bone ends with deeply impacted dirt are scrubbed and swabbed clean or trimmed with bone nibblers. Damage to the marrow cavity deprives the fractured ends of their blood supply and should be avoided.

Joints

If the capsule and synovium have been broached, the joint will require opening and meticulous cleaning. Tiny fragments of cartilage and bone are discarded, but articular surfaces should be restored as fully as possible. Immediate internal fixation to preserve congruity is the ideal, but with open contaminated wounds traction and early movement may be preferable. Occasionally, percutaneous wiring through clean skin may hold comminuted articular fractures together until early callus has formed or other fixation can be undertaken.

WOUND CLOSURE: EARLY VERSUS DELAYED

Two fundamental decisions must now be taken. The first concerns the timing of wound closure: the second involves the advisability of fracture fixation.

For small clean puncture wounds where the surgeon is satisfied that no debris or dead tissue has been retained, immediate wound closure allows primary healing. For wounds involving extensive tissue damage or retained foreign bodies such as the pellets from shotgun wounds or crushing, blast or high velocity missile injuries, the wound must be left open. They are packed with sterile dressings and are re-explored later.

Second and subsequent debridement procedures follow a similar pattern to the initial operation, but timing is very important and 3 to 7 days may elapse between operations. Infection, blood-soaked dressings or neurovascular deterioration are indications for earlier reassessment.

Other operations or fracture manipulations may be required under the same general anaesthetic. Between 48 and 72 hours muscle swelling and oedema are maximal. If closure at a second procedure is desirable, it is reasonable to wait for up to 2 weeks in order to allow skin suturing under minimal tension. The combination of inevitable muscle wasting with skin mobilisation by gentle undermining of fascia allows opposition of skin edges and closure. Indolent skin margins may be freshened with a scalpel blade to improve healing.

In contaminated wounds, suction drains or soft corrugated rubber drains can be inserted to the full depth of the wound and shortened daily under a rigorous aseptic technique. If closure has been premature and pus collects, the surgeon must not hesitate to reopen the wound.

FRACTURE MANAGEMENT – CONSERVATIVE VERSUS OPERATIVE TREATMENT

The major decision for all compound fractures concerns the advisability and timing of bone fixation. In ancient times various crude splints were employed. More recently Plaster of Paris became routine treatment (Fig 13.5).

Arbuthnot Lane introduced the bone plate and screws for fracture fixation and Kuntscher the intramedullary nail. The Swiss AO group has logically defined the indications and precise techniques for various methods of fracture fixation.

At first sight internal fixation might seem most appropriate for clean closed fractures where the risk of contamination is low. In contrast, open potentially infected fractures should preferably be managed by alternative methods.

However, modern theory now frequently advocates immediate internal fixation for the most serious open fractures as the bone fragments are then firmly controlled allowing better management of badly damaged soft tissues.

The challenge for the skilled accident surgeon lies in the selection of the ideal form of treatment for each fracture. For any single fracture the optimum treatment will vary according to the equipment available, the surgeon's experience, the facilities in the hospital, the adequacy of the nursing staff and the social and professional circumstances of the patient.

The surgeon must constantly balance the advantages of speedy recovery and early mobilisation against the potential risks of prolonged fracture fixation.

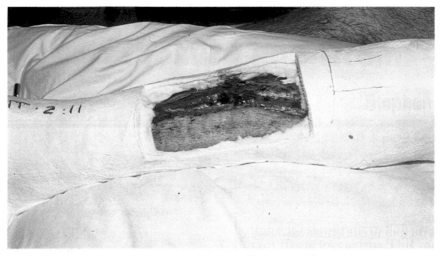

Fig 13.5 'Windowed' plaster of Paris.

Plaster of Paris

This represents the traditional method of fixation. It is easy to apply, easy to split, wedge, rotate, window or remove. Furthermore, it is strong, non-invasive and relatively safe. However, its disadvantage is that the joint above and below the fracture must be fixed thus immobilising the whole limb rather than the fractured bone itself. Plaster of Paris is not waterproof, obscures the wound and may itself cause skin problems by irritation and formation of pressure sores. Newer plaster materials have overcome most of these difficulties. They are lighter, waterproof, better ventilated and are radiolucent rather than radio–opaque. They are also faster setting. However, they are certainly more expensive, have a limited shelf life and may be more difficult to apply.

Cast bracing

The development of cast bracing with a flexible hinge allows earlier mobility at the joints, thus reducing stiffening and muscle wasting. This system cannot be applied at the time of fracture, but only when the fracture is already reduced and is beginning to heal.

Traction

Traction is often useful in the initial management of open fractures. In children, skin traction is sufficient but, in adults, skeletal traction is preferable. A pin is passed transversely distal to the fracture and, in order to minimise transfixation of soft tissues, the os calcis, tibial tuberosity or olecranon are usually selected. Frames, slings or pillows are positioned to support the limb and need frequent adjustment. The more complex the method of traction, the more essential are careful adjustments. The advantage of skeletal traction is that it allows joint movement and access to the wounds and is, therefore, suitable for severe injuries. It confines the patient to bed, needs frequent readjustment and provides relatively poor fixation of the fracture itself. The pins themselves may be a site of infection.

External fixators

External fixators depend on the rigidity of an external rod with transfixing pins to hold the bone fragments. The pins are bolted, clamped or cemented to the external rods which may be single or multiple. Compression between bone fragments increases the stability of the system and may well promote more rapid fracture union. Manoeuvering of the bone fragments with the pins in place enables a perfect fracture reduction to be achieved.

Internal fixation

Internal fixation of compound fractures has been enthusiastically endorsed by many orthopaedic surgeons and a wide range of equipment has been developed. It has helped to avoid the so called 'fracture disease' with muscle wasting, joint stiffness, skin problems and disuse osteoporosis which so often follow with less aggressive modes of treatment.

Meticulous aseptic treatment is essential. With open wounds, surgery should be completed preferably within 6 hours of injury. Plates of stainless steel or the newer inert alloys are used with suitable cortical or cancellous screws. Anything less than a perfect reduction with compression is unacceptable. Early mobilisation of soft tissues and joints is then possible.

A wide range of devices and instruments has been developed and each has its specific use. There is no place for the casual approach or the occasional operator.

Intramedullary nailing

Intramedullary nailing is ideally suited to transverse fractures of the midshaft of femur and tibia and is occasionally suitable for other long bones. Double fractures may be fixed, but great care must be taken that the power reamer does not rotate the central fragment jeopardising its blood supply.

Intramedullary nailing should not be combined with plating at the same operation as the double insult to the blood supply may devascularise large segments of cortical bone. If adequate nailing is achieved, immediate weightbearing is possible and early trouble-free union is usual.

Kirschner wires

Kirschner wires of varying gauge may be used to stabilise a bone fragment temporarily while other fixation is applied or, on occasion, may be entirely responsible for preserving fracture alignment.

Wires are usually inserted in parallel pairs with a power drill. If crossed, they provide less control of rotation and do not allow compression. When left projecting through the skin, removal is simple but pin track infection is possible.

Tension band wiring

Loops of flexible wire may be used to pull fragments together, such as comminuted patella fractures. When combined with supplementary parallel Kirschner wires, this provides excellent longitudinal control of olecranon or malleolar fractures even when they are comminuted.

Other methods of internal fixation

Nylon encircling bands with locating plates are useful for oblique long bone fractures. Carbon fibre has been used for ligament repairs, but must be avoided in compound fractures due to the risk of suppuration. Carbon fibre reinforced plates are strong, lightweight and radiolucent and may provide an alternative to metal plates.

Electrical stimulation

Weightbearing or early use of a limb is well-known to promote fracture union and this may be mediated through an effect on local electrical potentials. Electrical stimulation has now been adapted to promote fracture union either by inserting electrodes directly into the fracture site or by producing a local magnetic field with external coils. Used at present largely for patients with chronic non-union, the technique is rarely required in units providing good initial treatment.

Amputation and re-implantation

Improvements in vascular and plastic surgery have made amputation less frequent. While traumatic amputation often damages the parts beyond recovery, clean transection raises the possibility of re-implantation. This is most commonly attempted in the upper limb. Apart from the reattachment of an entire hand or arm, it is now generally accepted that re-implanatation should be performed for thumbs, for one or more fingers if all have been amputated and, perhaps, for the ring finger in women. The surgeon must be aware constantly that he is committing the patient to a long and arduous course of treatment. Serious cold intolerance is a complication which occasionally requires amputation of the reimplanted part.

Two teams of surgeons are preferred to prepare the amputated part and the region to which it is to be reattached. The bones should be fixed first and then the arteries and veins, followed by the tendons, nerves and skin. The provision of adequate venous drainage is always a problem and twice as many veins as arteries should be anastomosed. If there is any question of tension at the suture line, a free vein graft is preferable to bridge the gap.

Chapter 14

Wounds involving Major Blood Vessels
Averil O. Mansfield and John W. P. Bradley

Injury to major arteries or veins occurs commonly in patients with penetrating wounds or major fractures. Even the most innocuous surface wound may conceal serious derangement of important blood vessels beneath.

RECOGNITION OF MAJOR VESSEL INJURY

1 This may present itself as overt arterial haemorrhage in which case its control will require urgent measures second only in urgency to airway problems.

2 By evidence of interruption of blood supply to more peripheral structures (Fig 14.1). This may initially only be evident as pallor but will progress, if unrecognised, to pain and eventually numbness and loss of movement. These latter signs may be confusing if there is accompanying nerve damage.

3 By loss of pulses in the periphery. This is the most valuable sign and examination of peripheral pulses should be routine in every patient, but is essential when there are limb fractures or major trauma without fracture. It is especially important in the unconscious patient.

Notes on recognition
The presence of pulses should not be taken as an indication that there is no arterial injury, as it is possible to have partial interruption of an artery with distal pulses maintained. It is also possible to have a faint distal pulse produced by adequate collateral circulation, but comparison with the normal limb will usually confirm that pulsation is reduced. In spite of this, the absence of pulses remains the most important sign of the presence of an arterial

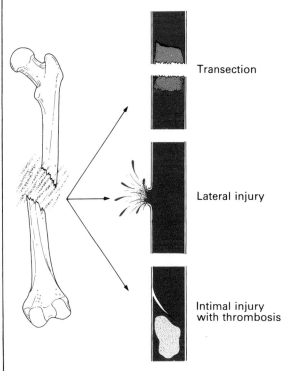

Transection

Lateral injury

Intimal injury with thrombosis

Fig 14.1 Causes of interruption of arterial supply.

wound and such a finding should initiate urgent steps to correct the abnormality.

INVESTIGATIONS

Arterial wounds are frequently associated with fractures of the long bones and a plain x-ray is essential in order to demonstrate the fracture site. The arterial injury site will be almost invariably at the same level as the site of the fracture, but difficulties may arise when two fractures are present to know which of the two is the cause of the arterial injury. The site of arterial injury in penetrating wounds, e.g. knife or gunshot wound, is usually self-evident, but blunt trauma can also produce arterial damage by an intimal tear which is more difficult to locate.

Arteriography

This is not always necessary and, indeed, in the vast majority of limb fractures associated with arterial injuries it simply delays the essential reconstructive arterial surgery. Similarly, penetrating wounds with a well established point of entry should not require arteriography for confirmation. If, however, there is a doubt about the presence of an interruption of arterial supply, or uncertainty as to its site, then arteriography may well be helpful (Fig 14.2). Care needs to be taken in interpretation of the arteriograms as the vessel may either thrombose or muscular arteries may constrict for a considerable distance proximal to the site of injury. If the injury is suspected of being in the thoracic aorta, confirmation of the injury will allow adequate preoperative preparation of the patient for a major thoracic procedure.

Doppler ultrasound

This mode of examination of the arterial tree is now readily available in most district general hospitals and may be of considerable value in trauma. It must be used with caution. The

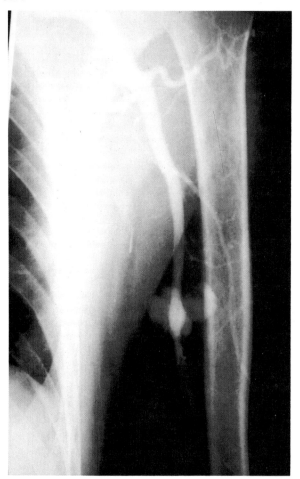

Fig 14.2 Angiography of the left brachial artery showing a false aneurysm after a stab wound of the upper arm.

presence of a doppler signal in a distal (e.g. pedal) vessel which has no palpable pulse should not lull the surgeon into a false sense of security. It merely indicates that the distal vessel is patent and measurement of the pressure in it, employing a calf cuff, is necessary to determine whether there is normal flow. Ideally, pedal pressure should be compared with brachial pressure, as the ankle/brachial systolic pressure index, and normally it should be 1. Any ratio less than 0.9 should be regarded as suspicious and a ratio less than 0.5 diagnostic of interruption of blood supply either from trauma or pre-existing arterial pathology.

MANAGEMENT

Restoration of arterial supply is a matter of some urgency and should not be delayed longer than is essential. Once the diagnosis has been made, exploration of that artery should be carried out immediately.

Where an associated fracture is present, it may be necessary to stabilise the fracture before undertaking arterial repair. If this fracture stabilisation is likely to take some time, then intraluminal shunting of the artery and associated venous injuries should be carried out first in order to lessen the period of ischaemia prior to restoration of flow on a permanent basis.

Temporary intraluminal shunting of major arteries and veins has been advocated by Barros D'Sa in Belfast in the management of limb trauma involving vessels, particularly the popliteal vessels. Several types of shunt are available and are used principally in carotid artery surgery. Most are tapered and have an expansion situated about 1 cm from the end. The wider end is placed in the proximal vessel and a specially designed clamp is placed distal to the expansion, thus holding it securely in the artery. Similarly, the distal vessel is cannulated after the shunt has been filled with blood and a clamp secures it in place (Fig 14.3). The Javid shunt is widely available, but has no side arm. The Brenner shunt has a similar design but with the advantage of a side arm for flushing and checking flow. The Pruitt Inahowa shunt has balloons at both ends to retain it within the lumen.

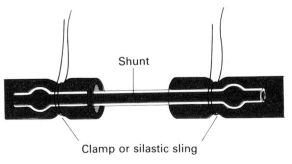

Shunt

Clamp or silastic sling

Fig 14.3

It is as equally important to cannulate and shunt the vein as it is the artery, because venous occlusion can jeopardise the survival of the limb, particularly when the injury is at the popliteal level. Once the operative site has been rendered stable, then the artery should be formally explored and exposed.

Complete transection
This is easily diagnosed at operation and the two ends of the artery may well have separated by some distance. The vessel will frequently spontaneously seal itself by thrombosis. The two cut ends should then be trimmed back to normal healthy artery. Although this may increase the gap between the arterial ends, it is an essential step and it is often possible, by mobilisation of the two ends of the artery, to achieve approximation of the two ends in spite of the loss of some arterial tissue. Bone shortening has sometimes taken place as a result of injury, or its stabilisation, and this can be advantageous in approximating the vessel ends. If a direct anastomosis cannot be achieved without tension, then the interposition of a vein graft becomes essential. The use of prosthetic materials must be avoided and it is exceedingly rare not to be able to find a suitable segment of vein to replace an artery.

End-to-end repair of the artery is achieved by placing two or three sutures equidistant from each other and completing the anastomosis with continuous sutures (Fig 14.4a). It is important to avoid narrowing the lumen, hence the necessity for at least two separate sutures so that the vessel can be stretched to its full diameter while the suture line is completed. This is particularly important when Prolene® is to be used in the repair because it slides through the tissues so easily that it is possible to 'gather', the artery and narrow it.

Incomplete transection
It is not easy to make rules about the way in which an incomplete transection of the artery should be dealt with. If the injury is a neat incision into the artery then it can often be repaired. If, however, there is extensive dam-

age to the area and a ragged wound, it may well be best to excise the segment and perform an end-to-end anastomosis, or excise part of the vessel wall and repair it with a vein patch.

Extensive damage to the artery with separation

Under these circumstances there is no alternative but to use vein in order to replace the injured artery: a reversed segment of saphenous vein taken from the uninjured limb is satisfactory and two end-to-end anastomoses are performed.

Intimal tear or subintimal haematoma

This is one of the most difficult injuries to diagnose because, externally, the artery may look completely normal or, at most, just slightly bruised (Fig 14.6b, pp. 136). There is complete interruption of flow through that segment of artery and diagnosis is often not possible until the vessel has been opened. The intima is lifted off by the flowing blood and a dissection ensues so obliterating the lumen. This event is best treated by excision of the damaged segment until normal healthy artery is reached, when an end-to-end anastomosis or an inter-position of a vein graft can be performed (Fig. 14.4b).

Technique of vein graft replacement of injured artery. Saphenous vein is the ideal material for replacement of the femoral or popliteal artery. Frequently, however, when one of these vessels is damaged so, too, is the vein. Under these circumstances it is unwise to use the saphenous vein from the injured leg and the opposite leg should provide the vein for grafting. If the saphenous vein is inadequate, it is almost always possible to find an alternative source of vein, e.g. the arm. The authors have never resorted to the use of prosthetic material because the potential risk of infection is too great.

An adequate length of vein is excised and its tributaries ligated flush with the vein. The vein is reversed and flushed through. If a long vein graft is needed, it is advisable to complete the proximal anastomosis first so that flow through the vein can be checked and twists eliminated. The distal anastomosis is then completed. Each anastomosis is formed using two or three separate sutures, as described for a direct arterial repair. If one anastomosis is obviously going to be more difficult because of access, then it may be advisable to complete this one first, even if it is the distal one, because freedom to manipulate the un-attached vein makes the anastomosis easier to complete. If the vein graft is to cross a joint, then it is important to assess the length of vein required with the joint fully extended.

Technique of vein patch (Fig 14.4c). When part of the wall of the artery has been damaged and excised, it can be replaced with a suitably tailored patch of saphenous vein. The patch should be only slightly wider than the defect as the object of the patch is to avoid stenosis and dilatation is to be avoided. The patch is tethered with sutures at two or three points and the suture lines completed with continuous sutures.

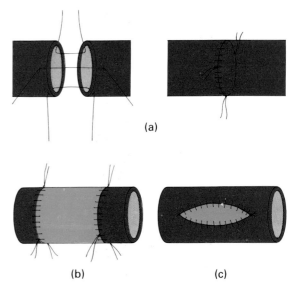

Fig 14.4 Methods of repair. (a) End-to-end anastomosis by triangulation; (b) vein interposition; (c) vein patch.

Additional features of management

Associated venous injury

When possible, any associated injury to the veins should be repaired. This is normally straightforward when a major artery, such as the femoral artery, is transected and the vein can usually be repaired by end-to-end anastomosis. It becomes of increasing importance when the popliteal vein is interrupted, as failure to repair the popliteal vein is the commonest cause of failure to succeed with popliteal artery injuries. If there is inadequate vein to carry out end-to-end anastomosis, then the saphenous vein from the uninjured limb should be used to overcome this gap, and it may be necessary to form a composite venous graft in order to obtain a sufficiently large vein to match the injured vein. In a composite vein graft, the vein is laid open by a longitudinal incision and a similar segment of vein is sewn to it, so forming a vein of double the lumen (Fig 14.5).

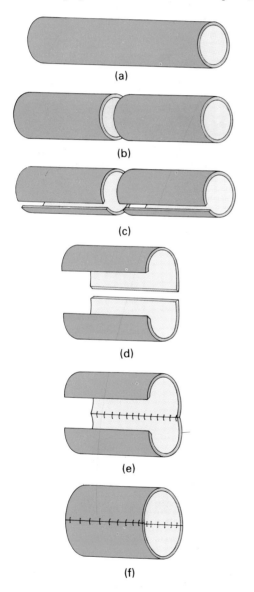

Associated nerve injury

Need for fasciotomy. Whenever popliteal arteries and veins are injured, a fasciotomy should be regarded as the normal requirement after the repair. This must include all compartments of the lower limb and one recommended method of carrying this out is the removal of a segment of the fibula. Three compartment fasciotomies may fail to decompress the central compartment, but are usually satisfactory. Fasciotomy under these circumstances needs to be carried out immediately after the repair has been completed, otherwise delay may result in irreversible damage to tissue. Vascular injury other than to the popliteal may also require fasciotomy, especially if there has been delay. It is better to err on the side of fasciotomy when there is doubt about its necessity.

Closure of defects

A lesson frequently relearned from war experience has been the fact that it is not necessary to close contaminated wounds; indeed, it is undesirable. In spite of this, it is desirable to cover a recently repaired artery and vein and so, although the wound may be left open, the repair should be covered whenever possible, even if this necessitates rotating a muscle flap in order to do so. Secondary closure of the wound or, if necessary, skin grafting may be carried out at a later stage.

Fig 14.5 Composite vein graft.

Infection

Suitable prophylaxis should be advised for the prevention of tetanus, and in contaminated wounds a broad-spectrum antibiotic is probably advisable.

Other drugs. Although anticoagulation is not normally advised in extensive injuries, one of the commonest complications of trauma is venous thrombosis and, following any extensive trauma involving vessels, subcutaneous heparin 5000 units 8-hourly for 5 days may be given.

RESULTS

In all arterial injuries one should expect to be able to restore distal pulses. If this does not occur, then a reason for this must be sought with urgency; possible reasons are distal embolisation or a second injury. The majority of patients having arterial injury are otherwise normal so far as their vascular tree is concerned, and a good result with distal pulses should be anticipated. Nothing less should be accepted.

COMPLICATIONS

The major anxiety in trauma surgery is one of infection, and the possibility of secondary haemorrhage from an infected arterial repair is always present, hence the need for prophylactic antibiotics. If secondary haemorrhage occurs, then it is likely that it will be necessary to ligate the artery.

Reactionary haemorrhage (Fig 14.6c).

This is almost always due to a technical failure and when haemorrhage occurs from a recently repaired vessel, it is a simple matter to correct the abnormality in most cases.

Compartment syndrome

This can normally be prevented by anticipating that it may be a problem and carrying out

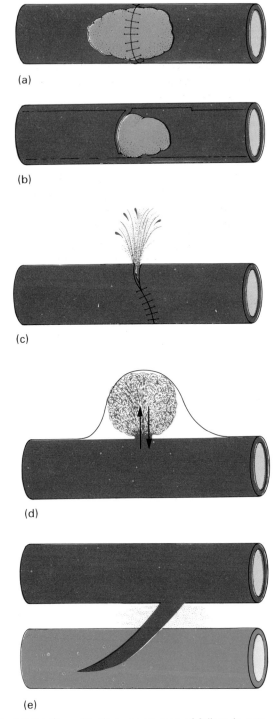

(a)

(b)

(c)

(d)

(e)

Fig 14.6 Complications or causes of failure in arterial injury. (a) thrombosis; (b) unrecognised intimal injury; (c) 'reactionary' haemorrhage; (d) false aneurysm; (e) arterio-venous fistula.

a fasciotomy. If a fasciotomy has not been performed, it is essential to observe the distal part of the limb with regularity and, if concern occurs about tension in one of the compartments, it is better to undertake fasciotomy than to wait and see.

Venous thrombosis

It is not easy to maintain the patency of a venous repair. Many investigators into this problem believe that the important period for maintaining venous patency is the first 24–48 hours and that if subsequent thrombosis were to occur, it would not be as important (Fig 14.7). Even when there is no venous injury, there is considerable risk of thrombosis and prophylactic subcutaneous heparin is advisable.

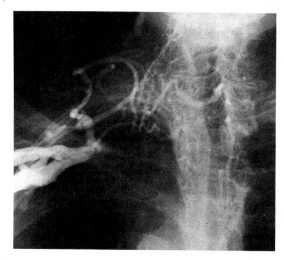

Fig 14.7 Venography showing thrombosis and occlusion of the left subclavian vein following a penetrating wound in the supraclavicular fossa.

Chapter 15

Penetrating Wounds of the Chest and Abdomen

Stephen Westaby

Deliberately inflicted penetrating wounds to the chest or abdomen are an increasingly frequent occurence in our violent society.

It is unrealistic to separate wounds of the chest from abdominal wounds since a large part of the upper abdominal viscera is contained within the bounds of the thoracic cage and knives or bullets frequently traverse both pleural and peritoneal cavities. Also the immediate management of patients with penetrating trauma is the same in each case: first, effective cardiopulmonary resuscitation and secondly, or simultaneously if possible, examination of the patient to formulate the sequence of the diagnostic manoeuvres to be followed.

Priorities in resuscitation are the establishment of an airway (A) via manipulation of the jaw or tongue, and intubation with a short airway, endotracheal tube or tracheostomy. Correction of the mechanics of breathing (B) then follows, by relief of tension haemo- or pneumothorax or covering a sucking chest wound. Third, cardiovascular (C) derangement must be assessed and corrected by pressure control of external haemorrhage, restoration of circulating blood volume or relief of cardiac tamponade.

This A,B,C sequence of resuscitation is an easily remembered and universally applicable process which must be instigated at the site of injury by the paramedical team. It is a useful rule never to remove knives or other transfixing missiles until the patient reaches the operating theatre and then only with direct access to potentially injured great blood vessels and, preferably, with the support of an autotransfusion system. Once in the accident centre, A, B and C are reviewed and a brief, but thorough, history obtained from the patient, witnesses or a police officer. The time of injury, type of weapon and condition of the victim during transport are noted. Nursing and medical staff remove the victim's clothes and evidence for future forensic or medico-legal investigation must be carefully preserved. Orientation of the garment on the patient, traces of gunpowder and missile fragments may constitute important parts of evidence and even tissue debrided from the wound edges should be retained. Physical examination must be thorough. The site of entry and exit wounds provides important clues to possible visceral injury and their size may reveal the kinetic energy of the missile and the extent of internal disruption.

The vital signs — pulse and respiratory rate, blood pressure and central venous pressure — are obtained. The last is of particular importance since the young and fit compensate well by vasoconstriction after blood loss so that blood pressure is maintained until critical hypovolaemia and acidosis occur. Blood loss is revealed by a low central venous pressure, though false positive elevation occurs with cardiac tamponade, shivering, straining or poor position of the catheter. To ensure an accurate reading, the catheter is inserted via the subclavian or internal jugular vein and an attempt made to make the patient relax and take a deep breath. At least two other large bore intravenous catheters should also be inserted for rapid volume replacement. A Ryles tube inserted by cut down in the antecubital fossa, then passed centrally to the subclavian vein, provides an excellent route for rapid, pressurised infusion and central venous pressure measurement if massive blood loss is anticipated during surgical intervention.

Decreased or absent breath sounds, subcutaneous emphysema, tracheal displacement, chest wall disruption with paradoxical movement, and neck vein distension are sought. Ventilatory support is initiated if respiratory efforts are inadequate or obstructed. Peripheral pulses are checked and the presence of bruits sought in the neck. In the presence of hypotension a radial, brachial or femoral arterial line assists accurate pressure measurement, blood gas and acid base determination. Once the intravenous lines are inserted, blood is obtained for haematocrit, blood grouping and cross match. Plasma volume expanders may be used initially but, with massive blood loss and persistent haemorrhage, uncrossmatched blood (preferably group 0 rhesus negative) must be used to preserve adequate oxygen carrying capacity and coagulation.

When the requirements of resuscitation have been achieved, a stable state is maintained by constant vigilance, continued assessment of the cardiovascular performance and adequacy of ventilation.

MANAGEMENT OF THE CHEST INJURY

Penetrating chest injuries frequently require prompt life-saving intervention by relief of tension pneumothorax, drainage of haemothorax or relief of tamponade on the basis of clinical assessment and before resort to chest x-ray or further investigation. Such procedures must be undertaken decisively and with confidence. The possibility of injury to the heart or great vessels must be considered,

however unlikely, since it is the unexpected rather than the obvious which most often causes disaster. When there is no exit wound in the chest, an abdominal injury may coexist. When the patient is haemodynamically stable, an upright chest x-ray (preferably postero-anterior) is obtained in full inspiration. The patient may require physical support and care must be taken not to disconnect the various catheters, since air embolus may occur on inspiration in the presence of low venous pressure. Supine x-rays are of little value in the assessment of intrapleural haemorrhage, airway damage, or co-existence of abdominal injury. Somtimes there is surprisingly little abnormality, especially when direct injury to the mediastinum leaves the pleural cavities unscathed. Mediastinal air, subcutaneous emphysema, pneumothorax and pneumopericardium are good evidence for injury to the bronchial tree or lung parenchyma. Haemopneumothorax is the commonest finding after penetration of the pleural cavity (Figs 15.1a; 15.1b). Heart size may prove deceptively normal in the presence of cardiac laceration and tamponade (Fig 15.1c), and should not cast doubt on the clinial diagnosis in the presence of circulatory collapse with high venous pressure. Widening of the mediastinum occurs after damage to the major vessels.

Decision making in penetrating chest wounds

Patients with spontaneous ventilation and stable haemodynamics

In patients with normal haemodynamics without respiratory distress and where the chest x-ray is normal, the patient may be kept under observation and re-x-rayed in 2–3 hours. If the clinical history suggests deep penetration (and in all gunshot wounds) the patient must be admitted to the ward for a 24–48 hour observation period, even when the clinical findings are unremarkable. When the chest x-ray shows a haemopneumothorax, a large intercostal drain (size 28–36 French gauge) should be inserted to evacuate blood and

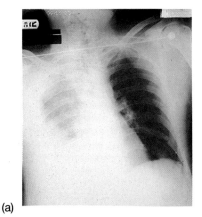

(a)

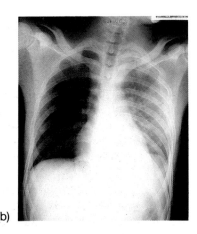

(b)

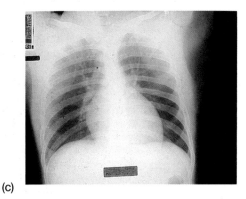

(c)

Fig 15.1 Chest x-rays in patients with penetrating chest wounds. (a) Stab wound of right lung and right atrium with haemothorax and cardiac tamponade. (b) Stab wound of left chest with wound of the right ventricle and cardiac tamponade. Blood had leaked through the pericardial laceration, but there was no injury of the left lung. (c) Direct parasternal wound entering the right ventricle with cardiac tamponade.

expand the lung. Usually one thoughtfully placed tube via the 6th or 7th interspace in the midaxillary line is the best initial approach. The tube is placed on suction and the initial blood loss and presence of air leak recorded so that subsequent drainage may be assessed. If the wound is several hours old, the blood will be dark in colour and initial drainage may be large because of the pleural effusion that accompanies small amounts of blood in the pleural space. The subsequent bleeding and the increasing or decreasing hourly trend is more important than the initial value and it is on this finding that further intervention is undertaken. A persistent air leak, especially in the presence of bleeding, and an incompletely expanded lung may indicate major pulmonary laceration, though this in itself is not an indication for further action in the stable patient. With blood transfusion and intercostal drainage, most pulmonary lacerations which do not directly involve a major vessel will resolve.

If any of the following are observed — arterial bruits, absent pulse , widened mediastinum or a wound track passing across the mediastinum — an aortogram should be performed to assess major vessel injury, bleeding from which may be deceptively controlled by a haematoma under tension. If the missile track crosses the mediastinum, a barium swallow and bronchoscopy are imperative, especially if mediastinal emphysema is seen on the chest x-ray or subcutaneous emphysema felt in the neck. If the entrance or exit site is below the nipple, careful abdominal examination and peritoneal lavage should be performed. When the chest tube drainage remains less than 150 ml per hour without a large or continuous air leak and if the diagnostic studies show no major structural damage to the trachea, bronchial tree, oesophagus or cardiovascular system, chest drainage and supportive measures are sufficient.

In some centres, there is an unfortunate practice of prophylactic chest drain insertion into patients with multiple injuries who require positive pressure ventilation. In the absence of blood or air in the pleural cavity and especially in the presence of pleural adhesions, there is a very real danger of creating a penetrating injury with pulmonary bleeding and air leak. The practice is, therefore, to be discouraged.

The importance of venous pressure measurements must be emphasised in patients with chest trauma since damaged lungs are very sensitive to overtransfusion and a brisk and inappropriate rise in venous and arterial pressure may reinstitute major haemorrhage in an otherwise controlled and stable state of hypotension.

Patients with unstable haemodynamics

These patients should be assessed carefully for signs of tension penumothorax (Fig 15.2), cardiac tamponade or major haemorrhage from cardiovascular injury. If tension pneumothorax is present, an immediate hole to release the air is the initial treatment followed by chest tube insertion when this is available. In the presence of an associated vascular injury, relief of tension may be followed by brisk haemorrhage as obstruction to venous return is relieved. When cardiac tamponade is present (Table 1), immediate periocardiocentesis should be performed followed by surgery regardless of the result (Fig 15.3). Time should not be wasted in applying ECG electrodes to the aspirating needle.

Early and effective control of the mechanics of ventilation is achieved by endotracheal intubation and intercostal drainage or covering

Table 1
DIAGNOSIS OF CARDIAC TAMPONADE

High index of suspicion	Site of wound
	Nature of weapon
	Direction of entry
Physical signs	Tachycardia
	Hypotension
	Venous pressure elevated
	Pulsus paradoxus
	Tachypnoea and anxiety
Investigations	Chest x-ray
	Two-dimensional
	echocardiography

of a sucking chest wall defect. Blood loss is replaced and further intervention determined in the light of clinical and radiological assessment. In Britain, where surgeons are less accustomed to penetrating chest wounds than in the US, there is a tendency to explore wounds more often to 'be on the safe side'. However, unnecessary exploration may change a relatively minor wound into a major chest injury.

As a result of large published experience of chest trauma from the USA and Vietnam war, we can formulate well defined indications for thoracotomy either on an urgent or delayed basis as follows:

1 If the initial chest tube insertion yields more than 1250 ml of blood immediately

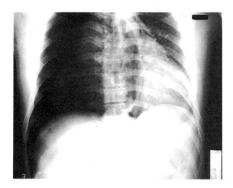

Fig 15.2 Chest x-ray of a tension pneumothorax.

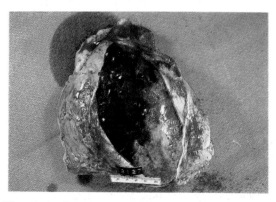

Fig 15.3 Postmortem specimen of a patient who died with cardiac tamponade. Note the bulging pericardium and clotted blood.

or more than 1000 ml plus 250 ml in the first hour, or if 250 ml is drained in 3 consecutive hours with no decreasing trend.

2 If cardiac tamponade is present, even if pericardiocentesis is negative or relieves symptoms.

3 For massive air leak where pneumothorax persists without adequate drainage suggesting a major bronchial or tracheal injury. Bronchoscopy is performed first.

4 In all transmediastinal wounds, aortography and barium studies should be obtained if the patient's haemodynamics are adequate and stable.

5 In most chest wall defects or diaphragmatic lacerations.

6 For removal of clot to prevent empyema. This should be considered after 48–72 hours of drainage. Enzymatic clot lysis is seldom successful.

7 For persistent massive air leak in the presence of an expanded lung after 7–10 days conservative treatment.

8 For combined thoracic and abdominal wounds (before laparotomy) except where entry and exit wounds preclude heart or great vessel injury or when the source of major haemorrhage is abdominal (Fig 15.4a–d).

In practice the most frequent indication for emergency thoracotomy is exanguinating haemorrhage via the intercostal drain, (from pulmonary hilar wounds) or tamponade from cardiac laceration. Occasionally immediate thoracotomy in the accident department may be life saving. However, since most patients have survived an ambulance journey to hospital, it is preferable to maintain a state of controlled hypotension, insert the appropriate lines for transfusion, correct acid base deficits

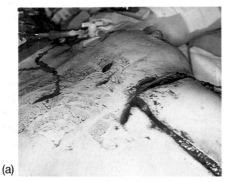
(a)

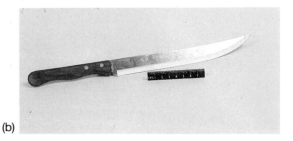
(b)

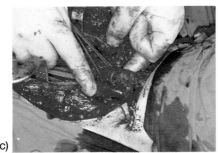
(c)

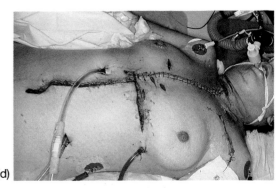
(d)

Fig 15.4 (a) Multiple chest and abdominal stab wounds. The chest wound lacerated the liver and spleen. (b) Weapon used to assault patient in Fig 15.4a. The length of the knife gave valuable clues to the extent of injury. (c) Stab wound of neck which transected the oesophagus and penetrated the superior vena cava and right lung. (d) The patient after repair of cardiac pulmonary, tracheal, oesophageal and hepatic wounds. The spleen was removed and chest and abdominal drains inserted.

and move quickly towards the appropriate facilities in the operating theatre.

At operation each individual injury is dealt with appropriately. Most bleeding areas in the ventricles or great vessels can be controlled with finger pressure (Fig 15.5). In the profoundly hypotensive patient, bleeding is minimal and once haemorrhage is stopped, blood or crystalloid infusion can be used to restore the patient's intravascular volume and blood pressure. If ventricular fibrillation occurs during thoracotomy, cross clamping of the descending aorta is a valuable manoeuvre. Cardiac massage then perfuses the cerebral and coronary vessels whilst blood volume is restored. Severe pulmonary laceration or contusion may require resection whereas cardiac, bronchial or oesophageal lacerations can usually be repaired by direct suture.

Large chest wall defects and sucking chest wounds require immediate cover to reestablish the mechanics of breathing. A sterile plastic wound drape such as 'Op-Site' is ideal for this and can be covered and supported by dressings and strapping until wound debridement and plastic repair are feasible. When an air leak coexists, it is important to allow air to escape, otherwise tension pneumothorax re-

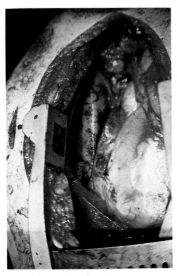

Fig 15.5 Median sternotomy adjacent to a right parasternal stab wound which penetrated the right ventricle and was successfully repaired.

sults. This is best achieved with an intercostal catheter inserted through a separate stab incision.

Gunshot or stab wounds below the nipple line may result in combined thoracoabdominal injuries and usually the abdominal component may be recognised by preoperative peritoneal lavage or examination of the diaphragm during thoracotomy. Diaphragmatic injury must be repaired carefully since the morbidity from strangulated diaphragmatic herniation is considerable. Formal laparotomy is preferable to a transdiaphragmatic approach, especially in the presence of vascular injury, a retained missile or suspected intestinal perforation.

MANAGEMENT OF PENETRATING ABDOMINAL INJURY

The airway, mechanics of breathing and cardiovascular status are again of paramount importance although A and B (*see* p.138) are unlikely to be seriously deranged in the absence of major blood loss or associated thoracic injury.

When the entry or exit wound is in the anterior abdominal wall, likelihood of intraperitoneal injury is high although, with stab wounds, deep penetration of the abdominal cavity is unusual, perhaps because the kinetic energy of the blow is low and the victim often has time to take evasive action. By contrast, high velocity injuries produced by gunshot or exploding shells may penetrate deeply, entering the abdomen or pelvis from an apparently innocent wound in the buttock or thigh and pursuing a bizarre course with extensive damage.

Apart from the history of the incident and superficial physical signs, the features which suggest intraperitoneal injury are concealed haemorrhage, peritoneal irritation or gastric stasis. Bowel sounds are only of occasional value since these may be absent in the presence of retroperitoneal haemorrhage and present in the presence of penetrating visceral injuries. Abdominal examination should pay particular attention to the presence of distension, localised tenderness, guarding, rigidity, flank dullness on percussion, and hyperaesthesia over the shoulder (Kehr's sign indicative of subdiaphragmatic irritation by blood). Abdominal girth is measured serially. Rectal examination is used to detect bleeding and abnormal swellings in the region of the prostate or lateral pelvic walls. Urine is examined for blood.

A chest x-ray is obtained in all cases, together with erect and supine abdominal x-rays where feasible. The chest film may reveal associated diaphragmatic or thoracic visceral injuries. Air under the diaphragm is diagnostic of rupture of an abdominal viscus. The presence of splenic or renal shadows is noted as is the outline of the psoas muscle which may be masked by retroperitoneal haematoma. The shape and situation of the gastric and colonic air bubbles may suggest a perisplenic haematoma, whereas a greyish ground glass appearance between loops of bowel may be evidence of intraperitoneal bleeding.

Four quadrant aspiration of the abdomen with a No.1 needle takes a few seconds only and may reveal copious free blood. If the result is negative, the more sensitive peritoneal lavage is performed by inserting a dialysis catheter subumbilically in the midline. When the peritoneum contains a large amount of free blood, this is immediately apparent. If the tap is negative or equivocal, one litre of normal saline is allowed to gravitate into the peritoneal cavity and the abdomen gently palpated to wash the fluid around. It is then allowed to syphon back into its bag. The result must be interpreted with caution, since false positive readings occur with traumatic catheter insertion. Injury in retroperitoneal structures such as the duodenum, pancreas or colon may be hard to exclude even with peritoneal lavage. When in doubt, the dictum 'it is safer to look and see than to wait and see' is more appropriate than for the chest, since a small perforation of an intra-abdominal viscus with

delayed sepsis carries a considerable risk of late complications and death. In practice, the decision whether to operate seldom requires more extensive investigation, though intravenous pyelography, selective arteriography and CT scans may have a role in certain cases. Movement away from the resuscitation area for such investigations must be undertaken with caution. Usually re-examination after a period of observation is of greater value in decision making and may avert a potentially hazardous journey to another centre with the required facilities.

One exception to this principle is in the event of potentially serious renal injury when an intravenous urogram is desirable to rule out unexpected pathology in the contralateral kidney which may profoundly affect the surgical approach. Unnecessary retroperitoneal dissection may either be avoided, or the appropriate splinting or drainage apparatus can be made available if such intervention is required.

When to operate on penetrating abdominal injuries

Definite indications for urgent or early laparotomy include:

1   Signs of massive intra-abdominal or retroperitoneal haemorrhage. It is desirable to transfuse and stabilise the circulation, except when blood is lost so rapidly that it is necessary to control the site of bleeding before resuscitation can proceed. This situation occurs when rapid infusion of 1.5–2.0 litres of fluid fails to produce significant improvement in the vital signs. Emergency surgery is undertaken through a relatively bloodless midline incision, preferably with the support of an autotransfusion system (in the absence of faecal, biliary or urinary contamination).
2   Other evidence of continuing blood loss, for instance through the wound itself.
3   Herniation of abdominal contents (even

when only a small tag of omentum protrudes).

4 Unequivocal signs of peritoneal irritation including local tenderness, guarding or rebound tenderness. Caution is required so as not to operate unnecessarily for a tender haematoma in the abdominal wall.

5 Free air under the diaphragm.

6 Unequivocal 4 quadrant tap or positive peritoneal lavage.

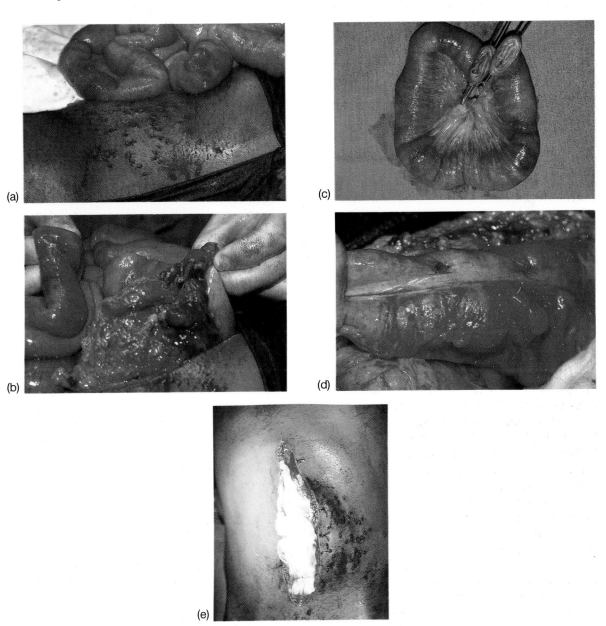

Fig 15.6 (a) Penetrating shotgun injury to the abdomen. (b) Perforated small bowel and haemorrhage in the omentum. (c) Small bowel resection to remove multiple adjacent perforations. (d) Colonic perforations oversewn. (e) Midline laparotomy wound with delayed closure of the skin and fat layers.

Patients not requiring immediate surgery are observed, the more seriously injured having a nasogastric tube passed to prevent acute gastric dilation. Continued monitoring of blood pressure, pulse rate, abdominal girth and urine output facilitate reassessment. Recent studies of a large series of stab wounds indicate that provided these rules are followed as many as 50% of patients will not require laparotomy, will spend a shorter period in hospital and more especially, have a lower morbidity rate. When warning symptoms and signs are acted upon promptly, no deaths are anticipated in those patients treated expectantly at first and subsequently requiring surgical intervention. It is probably wise to explore all gunshot wounds when there is reason to suppose that the peritoneal cavity has been traversed (Fig 15.6 a–e). The surface appearance of high velocity bullet wounds is deceptive and may conceal substantial injury.

A vertical midline incision is preferable in the emergency situation and is easily converted to a thoracoabdominal incision or extended in one or other flank to improve access to the spleen, liver or kidneys. Although, as a rule, it is desirable to excise a contaminated wound track and debride dead or damaged tissue, this is usually deferred until the end of the procedure.

Massive life threatening haemorrhage usually has an obvious source and is controlled initially by pressure or packing. Blood and clot is scooped and sucked out of the peritoneal cavity as completely as possible so that continued bleeding can be assessed. It is necessary to examine systematically every organ. A suggested sequence is spleen, liver, diaphragm, stomach, duodenum, pancreas, small bowel, colon, rectum, bladder and kidneys. Exploration of the retroperitoneal organs is especially important when the entry wound is in the back or buttock.

Damaged viscera are dealt with according to basic surgical principles, though recently the approach to damaged liver and spleen have changed. Splenectomised patients, particularly children, run the risk of overwhelming sepsis. Conservation with operative repair or partial resection are preferable except when speed is essential in the very shocked patient or when the spleen is hopelessly pulped. Similarly hepatic lobectomy carries a substantial operative and late mortality. In the acute phase resectional debridement proves safer, removing such hepatic tissue as has been virtually separated from the liver or has been irremediably damaged. When faced with difficult bleeding from the liver, it is sometimes wiser to leave abdominal packs *in situ*, drain the peritoneal cavity, then remove them 48 hours later when the bleeding has stopped. Alternatively, the vascular supply to the liver can be isolated by passing a shunt down the inferior vena cava from the right atrial appendage to below the renal veins. Snares around the cava first isolate the hepatic veins and then the portal vein and hepatic artery are clamped at the porta hepatis. Venous return to the right atrium is preserved via the intravenous shunt which reduces the risk of cardiac arrest in the hypotensive patient bleeding from behind the liver.

Chapter 16

Open Injuries of the Brain and Spinal Cord

Robert D. Illingworth

Whenever the coverings of the brain or spinal cord are breached as a result of injury, there is a serious risk of infection. This may occur in any wound in the body, but the consequences are particularly dangerous in the nervous system. The result may be meningitis or brain abscess, which can be difficult to treat and may result in permanent neurological damage. The outcome of missed or delayed diagnosis, and delayed or inadequate treatment can, therefore, be particularly detrimental. Open neurological injuries can conveniently be considered under the headings of (a) depressed skull fracture, (b) cerebrospinal fluid (CSF) leakage, (c) penetrating injury and (d) missile wounds of the brain. Wounds of the spinal cord and meninges will also be briefly considered.

DEPRESSED SKULL FRACTURE

As elsewhere in the body, depressed fractures are divided into those which are simple, in which the overlying skin is intact, and those which are compound, in which infection can enter through the broken skin. Many such fractures are due to road traffic accidents and are often associated with severe brain injury, as well as injuries to the trunk and limbs. The skull fracture may well not be a major part of the whole problem. Other causes are domestic injuries and assaults, and in these cerebral injury may be slight and other injuries absent.

If the injury has not broken the skin, inspection of the area will usually show only skin bruising and swelling, which will not allow any bony deformity to be felt. In compound injury the skin laceration should be inspected and, after cleaning, bone fragments or extruding brain may sometimes be seen. X-rays will be needed to confirm the clinical impression and show the degree and extent of fragment depression. Often the initial views will suggest greater depression than is actually present, and further views with the x-ray beam passing tangentially to the surface of the area of fracture will be required to give an accurate assessment (Fig 16.1a, b). Computerised tomography (CT) will show the degree of bone depression and also indicate any indriven bone fragments and underlying brain injury (Fig 16.2a, b).

For more seriously injured patients resuscitation, arrest of bleeding and airway care will take priority over treatment of the skull fracture. From the start, the usual principles of head injury management will apply, and careful monitoring and recording of conscious level, neurological signs, pulse, blood pressure and respiration should be done to detect deterioration due to the development of brain swelling or intracranial bleeding. CT or transfer to a neurosurgical department should be considered in patients with a severe primary cerebral injury with deep unconsciousness,

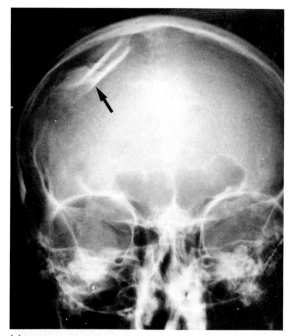

(a)

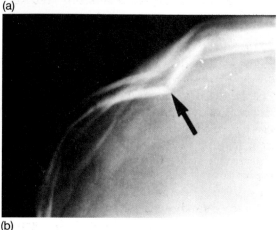

(b)

Fig 16.1 (a) X-ray of skull in AP projection showing depressed skull fracture.(b) The same patient with the x-ray taken with the beam tangential to the fracture showing that the true amount of depression is not as great as appears in (a.)

and in patients still not conscious after 6–8 hours. CT or transfer is mandatory in any patient showing deterioration in conscious level after admission.

Treatment

The hair should be widely shaved around any

scalp wounds and unless there is extensive skin loss the wound should be cleaned and closed in one layer with sutures. Large sutures inserted through the full thickness of the skin will stop any bleeding and this is easier and quicker than attempting to pick up and tie bleeding vessels individually. Provided the wound is closed, antibiotics started and tetanus prophylaxis given, no further surgical treatment to the fracture is needed for 24–36 hours.

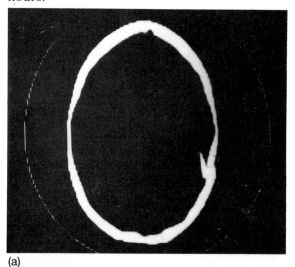

(a)

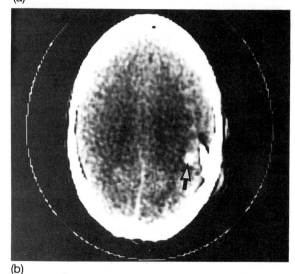

(b)

Fig 16.2 (a) CT showing depressed skull fracture in the right parietal region. (b) CT in the same patient with window level adjusted to show the underlying cerebral contusion.

It is a good general rule that all compound depressed fractures should be explored and elevated if there is depression greater than 0.5 cm, and particularly if the wound is contaminated with hair, dirt or debris. Another strong indication is the presence of separated bone fragments on x-ray, suggesting that the dura may be torn. Shallow fractures of 'pond' type may not need elevation if the wound is clean. Depression is not usually considered sufficient to require elevation unless the fragments are depressed by an amount equal to at least the thickness of the skull, or by 0.5 cm. Simple depressed fractures may need no treatment. The degree of depression is often not great and elevation is only indicated where cosmetic deformity will result if nothing is done. In infants, localised depression of the bone may correct itself over a period of time, but otherwise can be elevated easily and moulded back into place. The risk of epilepsy is not usually an indication for elevation. It used to be believed that a fragment of bone pressing on the brain may cause fits, but epilepsy is rare in closed depressed fractures and its occurrence is not influenced by elevation. Post-traumatic epilepsy is commoner after severe injury with post-traumatic amnesia of more than 24 hours, where there is tearing of the dura, and underlying cerebral damage.

Surgery should take place under general anaesthetic and be carefully planned. If the skin laceration is extensive or stellate, access may be gained to the fracture by extending the incision. However, if the laceration is small, or if extension would add to visible scarring, it may be better to turn a wide based scalp flap around the area. Care should be taken to keep a good blood supply to the flap by retaining the normal scalp arteries in the base of the flap and by not taking the incision close to the laceration distally. The base should not be narrower than the length of the flap.

Once the skin is opened sufficiently to show the whole depressed area, the pericranium is cut and scraped free of the bone. Fracture lines radiating some distance from the depression need not be exposed. All obviously dead or grossly contaminated skin and pericranium should be excised and any driven hair, dirt or debris carefully cleaned out. It is surprising how much foreign material may be found deep to a neatly sutured clean laceration. Although it is often possible to elevate the fracture by making a burr hole adjacent to the fracture and passing a lever beneath to lift it up into place, it is generally better and safer to lift the fragments out completely. Sometimes they may be mobile and easily lifted out, but more usually will need to be disimpacted by nibbling away a little bone with a small bone forceps before the pieces can be moved. Often the fragments include more of the inner than the outer table of the skull and some manoeuvring of the fragments may be necessary before they can all be removed. Alternatively, a formal craniotomy can be made with burr holes around the fracture joined by Gigli saw cuts to allow the depressed fracture and surrounding bone to be lifted out in one piece.

Once all fragments are lifted clear, the dura can be inspected for tears. If there is extradural blood clot, this should be sucked away, any bleeding stopped with diathermy, and the dura held up to the inner table of the skull with fine sutures passed through the dura and the pericranium around the bone opening to prevent recurrent clot formation. If the haematoma is large, or widespread, this last step is essential to prevent recurrence. If the dura is intact, but blue and bulging from underlying subdural haematoma, it should be opened and the blood removed by gentle suction. If the dura is torn, it should be opened widely and the brain inspected. All contaminated and severely damaged brain should be removed with fine gentle suction and all bleeding stopped with diathermy. In functionally important areas of the cerebral cortex, it may be better to be conservative in removing contused brain matter than risk adding to any neurological deficit. If there are any indriven bone fragments, these must be carefully sought and removed. Removal of all such fragments and debris, and meticulous haemostasis are essential steps to avoid delayed brain abscess or postoperative haematoma formation. If possible, the dura should be closed with small interrupted sutures. If not, a small defect should be closed with a patch of pericranium or temporalis fascia sutured in place, and a larger defect closed with fascia lata. Good dural closure is essential to avoid CSF leakage or brain herniation and artificial membranes are best not used in a contaminated field.

Traditionally, the bone fragments have been discarded but in most wounds explored within 24 hours in patients on antibiotics, this is probably not necessary even when there is contamination. The fragments can be carefully cleaned and fitted back into place after any trimming, which is usually necessary to get the pieces to fit. The aim should be to produce a tight fit and avoid mobility which may lead to bone reabsorption. Fixation with wire or sutures through drill holes is best avoided unless the fragments are unstable and displacement might lead to visible deformity, as in the forehead. Local antibiotic spray can be given and the patient should be placed on systemic broad spectrum antibiotics. Skin closure should be in two layers, with absorbable sutures through the galea taking any tension, particularly if there has been skin loss or the edges are ragged. If there is a little skin loss, wide undermining may allow closure but, if this is not possible, provision must be made in planning the procedure for a skin flap to be rotated to allow good full thickness cover over the fracture, and any defect which may result distally can be covered with split skin. A subcutaneous drain into a closed suction system will help to reduce postoperative bruising and swelling. Traditionally, the head has been covered after operation with a dressing of many layers of gauze held in place with crepe bandages. The author discarded this method many years ago and uses thin strips of cotton gauze held in place with adhesive tape for all operations on the head.

When a depressed fracture overlies the sagittal or transverse sinus, the question of elevation should be considered with caution.

Even if the sinus is not torn, elevation is likely to result in much bleeding and these fractures should not be elevated with a lever through a burr hole in case the bleeding cannot be reached and controlled. The fragments must be cut out and lifted free, and even then, if the sinus is torn, the bleeding may be difficult to control since patency of the sinus must usually be preserved. If the wound is clean and there are no fragments driven into the brain, it may be safer to leave the fracture unelevated.

Postoperative care

The subcutaneous drain can be removed at 24 hours, or later if drainage continues. Antibiotics are continued for 1 week and the skin sutures removed at 5–7 days. If there has been cerebral injury phenytoin 300 mg daily should be started and continued for 1 year. If any deterioration in conscious level or neurological signs occurs after operation, the possibility of intracranial bleeding should be considered and excluded by CT scan or re-exploration. If the bone fragments have been discarded because of contamination or infection, repair of the skull defect should be delayed for at least 6 months and should be performed with autogenous bone, such as split rib, rather than foreign material.

CSF LEAKAGE

Although this can follow compound depressed fracture of the skull vault, the usual causes are fractures involving the skull base and the paranasal sinuses. Leakage of CSF, often mixed with blood, may occur from the nose or ear and is usually obvious. Sometimes the leak may be slight or intermittent and may then be missed, especially in unconscious patients. If there is CSF rhinorrhoea, skull x-rays will often show fractures involving the anterior cranial fossa, the frontal sinuses or the supraorbital margins. Other basal fractures may not be readily shown radiologically even with tomograms, but bruising around the face, orbits or behind the ear may give an indication.

CSF otorrhoea results from fractures of the petrous bone and there is usually rupture of the tympanic membrane and visible leakage into the external auditory meatus. Occasionally the drum may remain intact and leakage will then occur via the Eustachian tube into the nasopharynx and be less easily detected, unless the patient is sat up with the head well forward.

Many CSF leaks will close spontaneously, particularly CSF otorrhoea, which rarely requires operative closure. Many leaks due to anterior fossa fractures will stop within a few days and this is more likely when there is little bone displacement. Leakage associated with displaced fractures of the middle third of the face is usually profuse, but stops after reduction and fixation.

The significance of CSF leakage is that it indicates a dural tear and fistula and this may also be indicated, without leakage, by the development of meningitis or the discovery of intracranial air, leading sometimes to an aerocoele (Figs 16.3a and b).

Diagnosis

Often CSF leakage is readily apparent, but this is not necessarily so, especially in the unconscious patient. It is wise to look for leaks actively in patients felt to be at risk because of the presence of a fracture or local bruising. The patient can be made to lie with the head dependent or to lean forward and cough in an attempt to provoke leakage. This may only occur intermittently and the patient should be given a bottle to collect a specimen which, if sufficient, can be analysed for sugar and protein. X-rays, as well as showing a fracture, may demonstrate opacity or a fluid level in frontal, ethmoidal or sphenoidal sinuses. Tomography in the coronal plane may give further help and in most patients with unilateral CSF rhinorrhoea it should be possible to decide the site of the fistula. If there is still doubt, CT with subarachnoid water-soluble contrast, or radioactive cisternography may be tried.

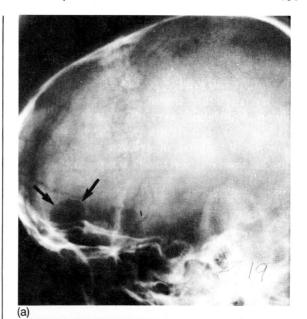

(a)

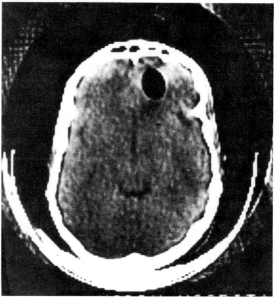

(b)

Fig 16.3 (a) Skull x-ray showing an aerocoele in a patient with an anterior fossa fracture and CSF rhinorrhoea. (b) CT in the same patient.

Treatment

Antibiotics should be given to all patients with CSF leakage, intracranial air, basal skull fracture, which might be associated with CSF fistulae, or with orbital or mastoid bruising.

The choice is between penicillin and a sulphonamide, or a broader spectrum combination such as ampicillin and cloxacillin. Nasal, or in otorrhoea, aural, swabs may help in making the choice and later, if meningitis is suspected, lumbar puncture should be done. Chloramphenicol, although very effective in penetrating the CSF, is best not used for prophylaxis because of the risk of aplastic anaemia, but can be reserved for use if meningitis should occur.

The indications for surgical repair are leakage persisting for more than 1 week, persistent or reaccumulating intracranial air or an attack of meningitis. Meningitis sometimes appears to seal a leak, but this is not reliable and multiple attacks of meninigitis may occur, sometimes over a period of some years. Sometimes profuse CSF leakage, through either nose or ear, may persist for years without meningitis resulting, but this cannot be considered an argument for non-intervention. Other indications for dural repair may be widely displaced basal fractures, perhaps with angulated bone fragments and meningitis, possibly years after a head injury, which should raise the possibility of a fistula. In contrast CSF otorrhoea nearly always ceases spontaneously and operative repair is rarely needed.

Repair of basal CSF fistulas is best done by formal craniotomy and intradural repair. The site of leakage is usually obvious from the skull fracture, especially if the leak is unilateral. If there is no visible fracture on x-ray, unilateral anosmia on the side of leakage may indicate that the cribiform plate is involved. Bilateral leakage suggests multiple dural tears, which are not uncommon in the anterior cranial fossa, or leakage into the sphenoidal sinus. Occult leakage from the ear into the nasopharynx can be suggested by deafness, and inspection of the tympanic membrane may show a fluid level or bubbles in the middle ear.

At exploration the site of leakage will often be shown by a tongue of brain passing into the fistula. This should be cut across and the defect patched intradurally with a piece of the patient's fascia; if small, from the temporalis fascia and if larger, perhaps to cover the whole anterior cranial fossa floor, from fascia lata. Suturing is not needed and simply laying the fascia in place with an overlap of 1 cm is sufficient fixation. Although anterior fossa fractures are often bilateral, careful consideration should be given before exploring on the side where there is no clinical leakage if olfaction is intact. Despite every care, it is only too easy to cause complete anosmia which is a significant disability.

Postoperatively the patient should be instructed not to blow his nose for 1 week and antibiotics should be continued for that time. If the leak persists or returns a search should be made for other sites and the patient re-explored.

PENETRATING WOUNDS

Most wounds in which the bone and dura are breached with penetration into the brain occur from compound depressed fractures. However, penetration can occur through small skin breaches which may be easily missed, and through small bone defects which x-rays may not readily show. These injuries can occur in road accidents from sharp projections on vehicles or from assaults with knives or tools such as screwdrivers. Another problem is the penetrating injuries which can occur through the orbit where the entry wound may be in the conjunctiva rather than the skin. These injuries usually occur in domestic accidents, often when a small child falls on a sharp object, or while holding scissors or a pencil. The injury may initially appear trivial and the possibility of penetration of the cranial cavity may not even be considered. Furthermore, x-rays may not demonstrate the defect in the thin bone of the orbital wall or roof, or through the ethmoidal air cells. The main risk is the development of a brain abscess, which is likely if the object is contaminated, and certain if contaminated foreign material has been left in the brain, as occurs if a piece of stick or pencil breaks off. X-rays will not demonstrate wood, but CT scan may show intracranial blood or air, or signs of cerebral injury.

When contaminated foreign material is known to have penetrated the head, exploration and the removal of all implanted material is mandatory. Where there is doubt CT may help and if penetration appears likely, exploration is advisable. If there is real doubt a compromise course is to use antibiotics in broad spectrum and repeat the CT scan in 3 weeks to exclude a developing, but as yet clinically silent, cerebral abscess.

Occasionally a neglected penetrating brain wound may lead to superficial infection in the skin and bone and the brain may then extrude to form a brain fungus. This needs antibiotic treatment and the control of intracranial raised pressure by drainage of any intracerebral or subdural abscess which may be present. If there is no intracranial infection, but the surface wound remains infected and unresponsive to antibiotics, the problem can be managed without operation, in expectation that the brain fungus can be controlled by lumbar puncture and that epithelisation of the mass will eventually occur. Excision should not be done since this is likely to lead to intracranial dissemination of resistant organisms.

MISSILE INJURIES OF THE BRAIN

This group of penetrating injuries includes those from gunshot wounds and missile fragments (*see* Chapter 12). The missile velocity is important since the amount of cerebral damage is much greater with high velocity missiles because the kinetic energy which is expended when the missile strikes is proportional to the mass of the missile multiplied by half the square of the velocity ($e = m \times v^2$).

High velocity missiles by their much greater energy produce damage beyond the immediate missile track and, though they may enter the head through a small wound, will often suck in debris behind them, scatter metallic and bone fragments at some distance from the track, and make a large exit wound from the head. The effect of this sort of injury is usually devastating and few survive a high velocity wound to the head. Unconsciousness is not always immediate, but rapid deterioration due to intracranial bleeding and massive cerebral swelling occurs, and patients deeply unconscious on arrival in hospital rarely survive. In practice, most missile wounds that survive to reach medical care in warfare are caused by shell fragments and the prognosis for these is much better than for high velocity bullets. Often these wounds are multiple and careful assessment may be needed to decide whether laparotomy or thoracotomy should be performed before the cranial wound is treated.

Low velocity wounds are more usually seen in civilian practice and, although the effects of a low velocity handgun bullet in the brain can be devastating, this may not always be the case. Airgun pellets can penetrate the thin skull of a child or enter through the orbit, but unless they pass through important areas, such as the basal ganglia and internal capsule, may produce little neurological damage.

Treatment

Treatment in high velocity injuries starts with resuscitation, control of bleeding and maintenance of the airway. Often respiratory obstruction or poor ventilation leads to rises in intracranial pressure, exacerbating the direct effects of the injury. Controlled ventilation and intracranial pressure monitoring and control with intermittent mannitol have become standard practice and should be initiated as soon as possible after injury. Early intracranial exploration may be required for control of bleeding, which can occur anywhere in the missile track and can be detected by CT, but usually debridement can be delayed a few hours until the patient is stable.

At operation the same surgical principles

that are used in the treatment of compound depressed fractures are applied. All destroyed brain, any indriven debris and bone and all accessible missile fragments must be removed. Removal of all bone pieces and foreign debris is important since delayed cerebral abscess is likely if any of these materials are left in the brain. A check skull x-ray after exploration is essential and, if retained bone fragments are seen, the patient should be re-explored. The risk of infection from metallic fragments appears to be less, and further cerebral damage should not be incurred by searching for fragments not easily accessible. Haemostasis must be meticulous to prevent postoperative haematoma formation. The dura must be repaired to prevent CSF leakage or brain herniation and, because of tissue loss, repair with fascia will usually be required. The bone at the margins of the skull wounds should be discarded and the defect closed later. Good skin closure may require a rotation skin flap if there has been extensive loss or if wide excision of devitalised tissue has been necessary.

Postoperatively ventilation should be continued for 48 hours, or for longer if the intracranial pressure remains raised at that time. Antibiotics should be given, and also anticonvulsants since epilepsy is common after these injuries. CSF leakage after a few days may indicate the development of hydrocephalus, which may require the insertion of a ventriculocaval shunt.

PENETRATING WOUNDS OF THE SPINE

The spinal canal may be transgressed by missile or stab wounds. The result is usually the development of a neurological deficit which, in the case of missile wounds involving the spinal cord, is usually complete and permanent. Occasionally, a stab wound may involve the spinal cord and produce a partial neurological deficit, often involving only one half of the spinal cord. In these circumstances, good recovery will often occur suggesting that the spinal cord has been contused rather than cut. In general, exploration of these wounds by formal laminectomy is not required unless there is evidence of wound contamination or if CSF leakage occurs. Antibiotics should be given and any skin wound excised if necessary and closed. Surgical exploration cannot be expected to restore cord function where there are clinical signs of a complete transection, but some benefit may occur in cauda equina lesions where prolapse of nerve roots through a torn dura can occur and the repair of this, with replacement of the roots within the subarachnoid space, may assist recovery.

Acknowledgement

Dr Hussein Abu Saleh, FRCS, Senior Neurosurgeon, University of Khartoum, Sudan supplied the information about brain fungus.

Chapter 17

Wounds to the Eye

Michael P. Quinlan

Injuries to the eyes occur frequently and represent the commonest cause of eye disease. The ocular tissues are delicate and injuries are potentially serious since they may result in blindness; elsewhere in the body trauma may produce only minor or temporary inconvenience. There have been few general surveys of ocular injuries, but a report on the range and extent of eye injuries in patients in Northern Ireland over a 10-year period found that blunt injury occurred in 49.2%, perforating injury in 48%, and intraocular or intraorbital foreign bodies in 8.4%. It was also noted that nearly one-third of adult eye injuries were the result of road traffic accidents.

ANATOMY

The eye is well protected because of its position within the orbit (a pyramidal space enclosed by bony walls), its cushion of fat and the intimate protection of the cone of extraocular muscles (Fig 17.1). Protection is also afforded by the blink reflex and lids and by the head-turning reflex on the approach of objects that are visualised.

EXAMINATION

Appropriate and prompt care of common eye injuries may prevent subsequent visual disability and, since they are often associated with other injuries that may be severe, it is important that the ocular involvement is recognised and the appropriate treatment carried out as early as possible. Neurological and faciomaxillary injuries need to be treated in conjunction with specialists in these fields.

It is essential that the vision is recorded with and without spectacle correction before any manipulation and, if necessary, with a pinhole to eliminate any refractive error. Many patients are unaware that their vision is defective either unilaterally or bilaterally and, if the vision is not recorded prior to the examination, they may subsequently claim that any reduction of it was due to treatment. Obviously, recording the vision is also part of the assessment and diagnosis of the patient.

A detailed history, where possible, is useful since it may help to indicate the type of injury, for example following hammering.

Both eyes should be examined including lids, lid margins, bony orbital margins, ocular movements, globes (for integrity), corneas, anterior chambers, pupils, lenses and fundi. Slit-lamp examination, where possible, is likely to be more accurate and fluorescein staining demonstrates any break in the epithelial lining. Care must be taken that the examination is thorough since occult perforation of the globe can occur even with a trivial injury. This is more likely to occur in injuries caused by narrow sharp objects such as darts, scissors and knives.

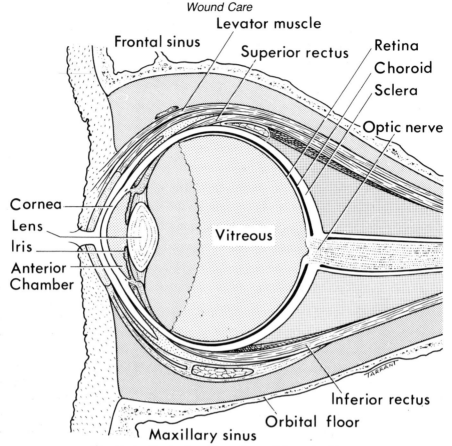

Fig 17.1 Sagittal section of eye, lids and orbit.

EYELIDS

Lacerations may be either horizontal or vertical or a combination of both. The depth of the wound should be determined and any foreign body removed. The bleeding can usually be controlled with suturing or cautery if necessary.

Horizontal lid lacerations are parallel to the lid margin. In superficial lacerations suturing is only indicated if the lacerated edges are gaping; if the laceration is deep, it may extend through the orbicularis muscle to expose deeper layers of the lid and closure should be done carefully in layers. Ptosis develops if the cut ends of the levator muscle are severed and not then sutured.

Vertical lid lacerations extend through the lid margin involving the whole thickness of the lid. Apposition of the edges is essential in repair to avoid a notch of the lid which is functionally and cosmetically unacceptable and subsequent scarring may give rise to cicatricial ectropion.

The technique of transmarginal lid repair involves three sutures across the lid margin. Various ones are recommended and used, but they are usually 6/0 or 7/0 in thickness. The first suture extends through the anterior aspect of the lid margin just posterior to the lashes, the second suture passes through the grey line, and the third suture goes through the posterior margin of the lid. The three-layer suturing technique should be performed for repair of full-thickness lid wounds.

Any injury around the medial canthus should be examined very carefully to determine whether damage or laceration has been sustained by either canaliculus. If one is torn, then the whole question of attempting patency by suturing the cut ends is debatable because the morbidity rate resulting from restoring continuity of the canaliculi is high. Lid laceration associated with facial lacerations and often with perforating injuries are most commonly seen following road traffic accidents.

Injuries to the lacrimal system in children have been classified into two groups. First, injuries to the nasolacrimal duct, usually associated with fracture of the orbit and lateral wall of the nose and including fracture of the middle-third of the face. Secondly, injuries to the canalicular system, most commonly avulsion injuries caused by hooks or dog bites (Fig 17.2).

CONJUNCTIVA

Lacerations of the conjunctiva usually do not require suturing since they heal rapidly. However, they may be obscuring an underlying scleral laceration and when there is doubt the conjunctival laceration should be explored and examined, under anaesthetic if necessary.

Foreign bodies in the conjunctiva, especially in the lower fornix, are usually washed out by themselves. However, subtarsal foreign bodies often need to be removed since they become embedded in the upper tarsal conjunctival surface. They can easily be taken out following eversion of the upper lid. They are extremely

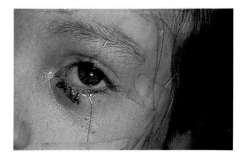

Fig 17.2 Lower lid laceration following a dog bite which involved the inferior canaliculi. The canaliculi have been temporarily intubated and lid sutured.

painful, especially on blinking, and are suspected when fine superficial corneal abrasions covering mainly the upper half of the cornea are seen.

CORNEA

About 75% of all ocular injuries involve the cornea and corneal foreign bodies account for about one–third of these. They are important since they constitute a risk to sight by corneal scarring with its subsequent blurring of vision and may cause irregular refractive errors by altering corneal curvature. Corneal foreign bodies are associated with the symptoms of pain, lacrimation and photophobia and it may be necessary to instil topical anaesthetic drops to make a complete examination. Removal of a foreign body is most effective with slit-lamp magnification and a hypodermic needle, but if these are not available it is worth trying irrigation and a cotton-wool tipped applicator. Complete removal of the foreign body encourages epithelisation and relief of pain. Topical antibiotics are applied and if blepharospasm, keratitis or uveitis is present, then a cycloplegic drop instilled topically relieves the associated ciliary spasm.

Corneal abrasions

These usually have a history of trauma which may have been minor (for example, the twig of a tree catching the eye) and symptoms of pain, lacrimation and photophobia. Instillation of fluorescein drops produces a corneal stain and the treatment is occlusion of the eye with a pad and topical antibiotic and, if severe, a mydriatic (Fig 17.3).

Recurrent abrasions may occur as entities or may be associated with corneal dystrophy. The patient has a history of an abrasion that heals and then, after a lapse of time, there is a sudden recurrence of symptoms on waking in the morning. An abnormal basement membrane or its lack of regeneration is one theory why basal cells detach readily after regenera-

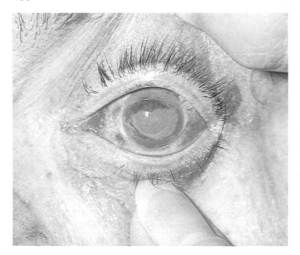

Fig 17.3   Corneal abrasion stained with fluorescein.

tion of an epithelial defect. It may be necessary to debride the affected area and to use topical ointment at night over a long period.

Corneal lacerations

Corneal lacerations, unless of puncture type, are often associated with iris prolapse and the pupil then has the characteristic appearance of a tear drop. There may be associated prolapse of ciliary body, lens and vitreous body or even retina if the injury is severe. Superficial injuries of the cornea are painful, but perforating injuries are often painless although they may be associated with shock (Fig 17.4). Once the diagnosis has been made in such an injury, no further investigation should be undertaken until the patient is examined under anaesthetic in the operating theatre with an operating

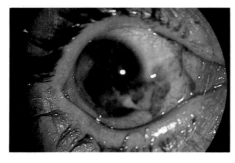

Fig 17.4   An eye with extensive damage including corneal laceration and iris prolapse.

microscope. In all such cases radiology of the orbit to exclude an intraocular foreign body is mandatory.

The wound may be self-sealing or may leak. Leaking can be demonstrated by instilling topical fluorescein into the tear film: a cascade of aqueous is seen if a leak is present.

Surgery of a corneal wound should aim at replacement of any prolapsed tissue that is still viable and excision where this is not possible, and then exact apposition of wound edges to restore ocular tension. The anterior chamber may be reformed with air if it has collapsed. A monofilament suture with buried knots prevents irritation and vascularisation and permits early fitting of a contact lens. Surgery should be performed with an operating microscope.

HYPHAEMA

Blunt injuries to the globe often produce bleeding into the anterior chamber. This does not clot, but forms a meniscus level which usually settles and is absorbed with conservative treatment. It has been found that in 134 out of 197 cases absorption of hyphaema occurred within 5 days with conservative management. However, a secondary haemorrhage may occur within a few days. Out of 289 patients with primary traumatic hyphaema, 27 developed a secondary hyphaema. With secondary haemorrhage there is a risk of associated glaucoma and this occured in all patients who had had a total secondary haemorrhage at some stage. Another complication is invasion of the corneal substance by blood corpuscles. When this occurs in association with a rise of tension, bloodstaining of the cornea may develop. However, the prognosis with this is good in the absence of associated ocular damage, although clearing of the cornea may take a number of years.

When the hyphaema has cleared, underlying damage may be visible. Trauma of the iris may produce sphincter paralysis with traumatic mydriasis (Fig 17.5); a tear of the

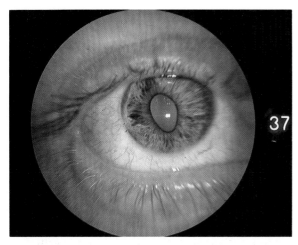

Fig 17.5 Traumatic pupil-sphincter damage producing an oval pupil.

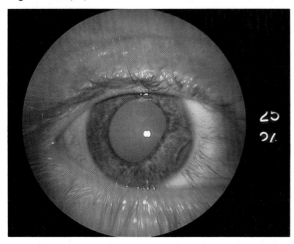

Fig 17.6 Concussion injury with iridodialysis.

iris margin has the characteristic notched appearance of sphincter rupture. Tearing of the iris from the ciliary body producing iridodialysis (Fig 17.6) or recession occuring at the drainage angle may give rise to subsequent glaucoma. It is important, therefore, to use gonioscopy to examine the drainage angle in all patients with traumatic hyphaema. A total hyphaema almost invariably accompanies every case of traumatic aniridia.

LENSES

Blunt or perforating injury to the lens may produce cataract. It has been shown that traumatic cataracts are initially subcapsular anteriorly or posteriorly and with time recede into the cortex. Intraocular foreign bodies may stop in the lens as demonstrated in Fig 17.7 and then the whole lens should be removed, or they may pass through it. If the anterior capsule is ruptured then the rest of the lens should be removed. This may be done by aspiration or a lensectomy performed with one of the infusion suction cutter machines. However, if the posterior capsule is also damaged, preservation of this should only be considered if the damage is not very extensive and there is no large vitreous prolapse. If vitreous is present in the anterior chamber, a more satisfactory result is achieved with total removal of the lens and partial anterior vitrectomy.

The lens, normally suspended by the fibres of the suspensory ligament, may become displaced; subluxation or complete rupture of the ligament may give rise to dislocation. Complete dislocation frequently leads to uveitis, pupil-block glaucoma and retinal detachment. In perforating injuries, where lens matter and vitreous mix, vitrectomy should be considered.

CHOROID

Contusion injuries directed to the choroid

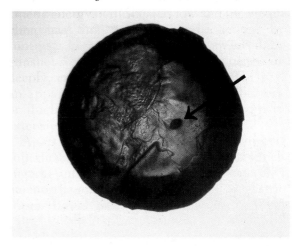

Fig 17.7 Intraocular foreign body within lens.

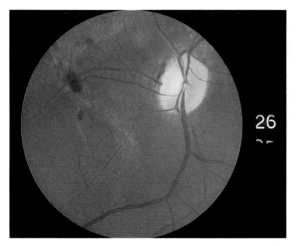

Fig 17.8 Fundus photograph of an old choroidal rupture with associated pigmented epithelial changes over the macular area.

produce choroidal rupture with a characteristic appearance and may be disastrous for vision if the macula is involved (Fig 17.8). Unfortunately, no treatment is effective.

RETINA

After contusion of the globe, the retina may develop commotio retinae (Berlin's oedema). Clinically, the picture is of a grey-white colour to the retina which may be confined to the macular area or may also involve areas of the peripheral retina. These changes have been attributed to photoreceptor outersegment damage. There may be associated subretinal haemorrhages and choroidal rupture. In some patients the macular changes may clear completely and central vision may be restored while, in others, there may be some loss of central vision with pigmentary disturbance and macular hole formation. Retinal detachments may arise due to retinal dialysis. It is known that 20% of all detachments are due to dialysis and ocular trauma is involved in the aetiology.

SCLERA

Scleral lacerations often extend to the cornea and there is associated prolapse of both iris and ciliary body. If the ciliary body is involved, then there is usually loss of vitreous as well. At surgery the full extent of the wound must be exposed and vitreous cleaned from the wound, and the laceration is then closed with interrupted sutures.

PERFORATING INJURIES

Usually the history suggests the risk of perforating injury even if it is not clinically obvious, for example hammering. Where there is such a history, x-rays should always be obtained. They are of value for screening for the presence of foreign bodies and also for their localisation (Fig 17.9). Ultrasound is also useful in the presence of foreign bodies (Fig 17.10). Radiological detection and localisation of foreign bodies is preferable to ultrasound, but the latter serves as a useful adjunct to x-ray localisation for measuring ocular dimensions and indicating associated tissue damage. Ultrasound techniques are the sole method of localisation of radiolucent foreign bodies. Metal detectors may also be helpful in diagnosis, especially when there are opaque media precluding a good view at operation.

Once perforation has occurred, the foreign body may stop in any ocular tissue along its pathway. It may still be lodged in the cornea or may have ended up in the anterior chamber where it falls into the angle and may only be visible with a gonioscope. It may penetrate the iris or lodge there, it may pass into the lens and settle there or go through into the vitreous, or it may miss the lens and pass through into the zonule. If it reaches the coats of the eye, the retina in the equatorial region is the commonest site in which it settles. However, it may penetrate the coats. The optic nerve tends to be soft tissue and it may pass into this and through and even out of the eye again.

Marked injury may occur to the eye as a result of concussion from a foreign body that never penetrates the eye. The site at which the particle finishes determines the extraction

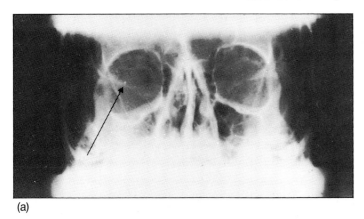

(a)

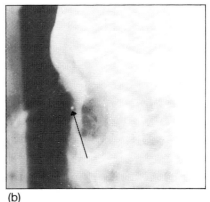

(b)

Fig 17.9 X-ray showing intraocular foreign body in the right eye on (a) anteroposterior view and (b) lateral view.

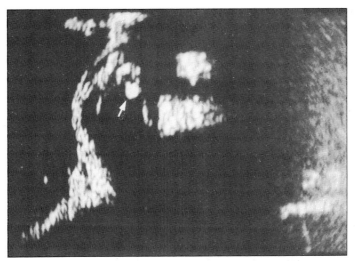

Fig 17.10 Ultrasound scan showing intraocular foreign body; the horizontal B-scan section on deviated gaze shows an intravitreous foreign body (arrow) on an attenuating sound beam.

route. If the particle is magnetic then a magnet can be used for its removal but, if non-magnetic, then instrumentation within the eye is necessary.

The prognosis for perforating eye injuries has improved, but this is mainly due to better results from anterior segment injuries. There has been little change in the prognosis for injuries to the posterior segment over the last 15 years. Traction retinal detachment is the main reason for visual loss in posterior segment injuries. However, new techniques and instrumentation for vitreous surgery are alter-

ing this position in the management of ocular trauma. Closed virectomy, usually through a pars plana approach, helps in clearing ocular media opacities, relieving vitreoretinal traction, removing intraocular foreign bodies, restoring aqueous flow and treating endophthalmitis complicating trauma. The optimum timing and indications for vitrectomy are, nevertheless, still controversial. One survey reported the histological findings in human eyes after severe penetrating trauma. The results indicate that a damaged lens, the admixture of lens material and vitreous, and

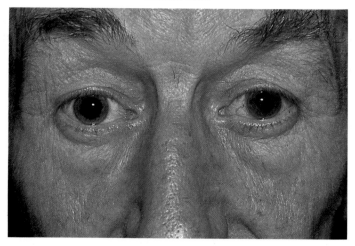

Fig 17.11 Both eyes of a patient with haemosiderosis of the left eye. This is demonstrated by the different colour of the iris, chronic uveitis and associated cataract.

the presence of vitreous haemorrhage were all factors promoting the proliferation of fibroblasts within the vitreous. The stimulus and scaffold for this proliferation were removed by vitrectomy which, it was suggested, should not be delayed beyond the second week of injury.

Certain foreign bodies may be retained with minimal reaction. Iron and copper, however, oxidise rapidly with resulting siderosis (Fig 17.11) and chalcosis respectively. The reaction to chemical activation from copper may be sufficient to cause panophythalmitis and rapid destruction of the eye. Other substances such as glass and plastic are inert and can be left in the eye with no reaction.

CHEMICAL BURNS

Chemical burns of the conjunctiva and cornea should be treated by immediate irrigation with copious amounts of water. Particulate matter should be removed from the surface. Acid burns are quickly buffered by the tissues and the immediate injury is the full extent of the damage, but in alkali burns the injury is aggravated as times goes on because of the continual release of hydroxyl ions into the tissue.

Alkali burns of the eye are among the most disastrous of ocular injuries since they characteristically result in blinding corneal opacification followed by intense vascularisation, chronic irritation, conjunctival overgrowth and persistent morbidity. Repeated ulceration or perforation of the extensively burned cornea is common. Contact lenses may be helpful in promoting re-epithelisation. Corneal transplantation may be indicated in the more severe cases, but the results are generally unfavourable due to poor healing and opacification of the cornea.

RADIANT ENERGY

With most forms of electromagnetic energy the degree of damage is related to the amount of absorption of the energy by the specific ocular tissue. Infrared radiation is transmitted by the cornea and lens and comes to a focus on the retina, for example in eclipse burn retinopathy. It is thought that the acute foveal lesion is caused by a photochemical injury rather than a thermal injury to the retina and pigmented epithelium.

Ultraviolet radiation is absorbed almost completely by the conjunctiva and cornea and produces a superficial punctate keratitis, for example in exposure to a sunray lamp.

X-rays, gamma rays and alpha and beta particles may damage any part of the eye and they all produce cataract.

THERMAL BURNS

Thermal burns are caused by flare or flame and usually result in widespread tissue destruction involving the lids rather than the globe. Splashes of molten metal or other hot liquid cause the majority of surface ocular burns. Thermal burns create ocular complications by contraction of coagulated skin, contraction of shrinking scar tissue in the later stages and resultant corneal exposure with the risk of corneal ulceration and infection. The corneal exposure is made worse by relative immobility of the lids and globe. Contact lenses, tarsorrhaphy, mucous membrane graft and plastic procedures to the lids are all helpful in treatment. The last may be done in conjunction with the plastic surgeon.

SUMMARY

Many of the ocular injuries could be prevented by simple measures: in industry, by wearing protection for the eyes; in road traffic accidents, by wearing seat belts; and in sport, by wearing protective clothing. From this article it is apparent that the surgical approach to many cases of trauma has changed within the last few years and the results have improved quite considerably.

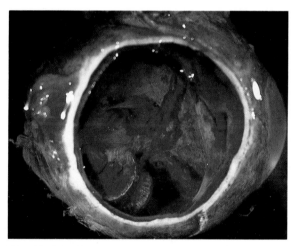

Fig 17.12 Hemisection of an eye enucleated because of severe injury showing an air-gun pellet lying within the eye.

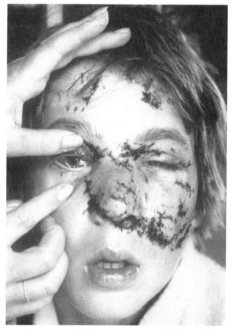

Fig 17.13 Typical injuries associated with a road traffic accident. There is a perforating injury of the right eye and extensive facial lacerations.

Chapter 18

General Treatment of Burns

Roy Sanders

Pain, fluid loss, infection and disfigurement are all factors to be considered when treating burns.

Certain circumstances expose people to a greater risk of accident and so a burnt patient often has a problem before being burnt, such as social deprivation, epilepsy, alcoholism, stress, psychosis, age or debilitating disease. The ability to cooperate with treatment may then be limited. Age, malnutrition and concomitant disease may render them more susceptible to infection and healing processes may be slower. Even a small burn should be regarded as a serious injury.

The way in which the burn occurred, if carefully noted, will give important clues as to the depth of injury. This is critical since a burn involving only the superficial layers of the skin, if properly managed, will heal without grafting. A deeper burn may require surgery. Burns of less than 10% of the body surface, although serious, are not associated with major fluid loss and disorders of metabolism.

Burns are classified as *superficial* (damaging only epidermis and superficial layers of the dermis); *deep dermal* (preserving only the deeper layers of dermis, hair follicles and sweat glands); and *full thickness* (where all of the skin, follicles and glands are destroyed).

Of all burns, scalds are the most common. They are often of limited extent and depth, and heal quickly with insignificant scarring, but they may be extensive and deep. The heat

of the liquid and how soon cooled are facts which, if recorded, guide in the diagnosis of depth of injury. Clothing soaked in hot liquid, if not removed or cooled, greatly increases the severity of burning (Fig 18.1). Flame burns almost invariably destroy the full thickness of part of the burnt area. If they result from ignited clothing, the front of the body, neck, face and palms of the hands are burnt. Conduction burns from electrical domestic appliances are always full thickness. Damage extends along vessels and nerves since this plane constitutes the line of least electrical

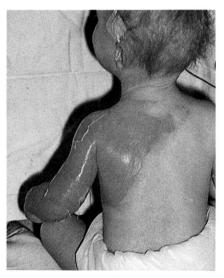

Fig 18.1 Scald from a spilt teapot. Deeper scalds resulted from garments retaining the hot fluid.

resistance (Fig 18.2). High tension electrical burns from power lines cause damage to the skin at entry and exit sites and extensive damage to muscle between the two points (Fig 18.3).

Flash burns from explosion of inflammable gases or vapours or the discharge of electricity are always partial thickness so long as clothing has not been ignited. Healing occurs in 10 days. Contact burns are very common at home. If the hand or other part can be withdrawn from the heat (a hand on the iron or oven door) the burn is always partial thickness. If trapped, for example, in a hot press of some kind, the burn is much deeper and may be associated with crush injury (Fig 18.4).

Chemical burns resulting from industrial accidents or assault are usually of limited

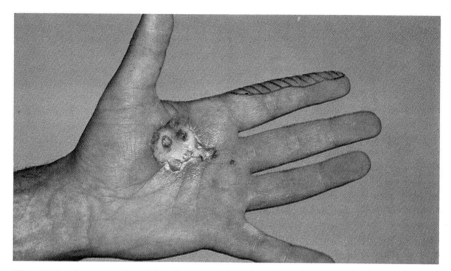

Fig 18.2 A conduction burn from a faulty electrical drill. The digital nerve of the index finger was damaged.

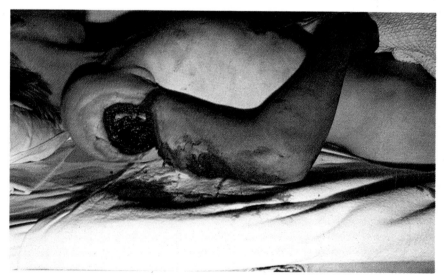

Fig 18.3 Gross tissue destruction from a high tension electrical burn. Extensive damage was done to underlying tissues.

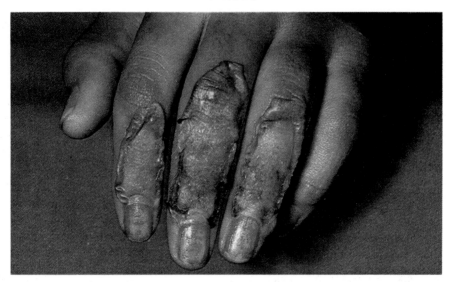

Fig 18.4   A deep burn from an industrial hot press.

extent and confined to the skin, unless the agent has been swallowed or the patient has been accidentally immersed. The depth of the burn will depend on the concentration of the chemical and whether it was quickly diluted by washing. Patients unconscious at the time of burning more commonly suffer deeper burns.

THE EFFECT OF BURNING

When skin is burnt its ability to protect against water loss and bacterial invasion is lost. Vessel permeability is increased and plasma is lost from the vessels into the tissue spaces and from the surface. Bacteria may proliferate in the tissues and spread, causing septicaemia. The effect of a burn arises from products of tissue destruction, the loss of water, electrolytes and protein, and the toxins of invading bacteria.

The aim of burn wound management is to avoid or limit bacterial invasion of the wound, to promote comfort and healing and to avoid any further damage to the healing tissues.

THE HEALING OF BURNS

Where only part of the thickness of the skin is

destroyed, the hair follicles, sweat and sebaceous glands remain. From these structures new epidermal cells spread between dead superficial dermis and the living, deeper layer to re-establish the epidermal layer. The process takes between 7 days and several weeks, depending on the depth of injury, the age of the patient and whether infection is present.

When the full thickness of the skin is destroyed, there are no follicles or glands remaining and epidermis must spread from the margins of the wound. This is an effective process if the wound is small but, if more than a few centimetres in diameter, healing may never occur, since the epithelial cells migrating from the margins must move over a base which becomes fibrous and unable to support them. Grafting is then needed.

MANAGEMENT OF THE BURN WOUND

To reduce pain and limit oedema in burnt and non-burnt parts, the burn should be cooled in water at about 20°C for at least 10 minutes. Ice, or iced water, if applied for long periods, may cause local damage from frostbite or result in hypothermia and should be used with

Table 1
FIRST AID TREATMENT

Superficial burns/scalds
Immersion under a running cold tap will reduce pain
The wound should be left exposed to the air

If clothing is alight
Extinguish flames with cold water or by smothering
Remove smouldering or soaked fabric where possible, but leave any which has cooled
Flood the affected part with cold water if possible
Cover with a sterile or clean dressing or cloth

Electrical burns
Disconnect power supply or remove patient from the power source using a wooden or rubber implement
Check respiration and cardiac output — resuscitation may be necessary

Chemical burns
Flood area with cold, running water continuously to dilute and eliminate the chemical
Carefully remove contaminated clothing, preferably under running water, without self contamination
Specific industrial antidotes may be available.

---

care. First aid treatment of burns and scalds is shown in Table 1.

There are various ways of managing a burn wound so that bacterial invasion and proliferation are avoided or reduced. No matter how the wound is treated, it is important to remember that there is a sensitive and anxious patient to consider; the treatment should not hurt or harm the patient in any way and the functions of joints and muscles must be preserved by physiotherapy.

Exposure and drying of the surface may be regarded as the natural way to treat a wound. Bacteria do not thrive in a dry environment. An eschar forms from the dead tissue and protein exudate and this eventually separates to reveal either a healed epidermal surface or a granulating wound. An exposed wound allows patient and wound to be observed without impediment and movement, feeding and bodily functions can be performed unhindered. Considerable heat and fluid loss occur.

Exposure is an effective treatment for a small wound on a surface which is easily exposed. If the burn is extensive and involves a surface on which the patient must lie, that wound becomes wet and infected. To limit this, continual turning is necessary, which is demanding of nursing time and skill, and often painful for the patient.

In many centres only the face is exposed and other areas are treated by dressings, plastic bags or by surgery. Dressings avoid some problems and create others. Access and observation are difficult. Heat and fluid loss are limited, but there is as yet no universally satisfactory agent to prevent infection beneath the dressings. Such measures are very costly both in terms of materials and staff. A dressing should be comfortable when applied, worn and removed. So, it should be soft and not too tight, but not so loose that it falls off. It should be absorbent of exudate and thick enough for fluids not to 'strike through'.

A non-irritating and non-toxic agent should be applied in the dressing to deter infection. The most commonly used materials are silver sulphadiazine (Flamazine®), providone-iodine (Betadine®) and chlorhexidine cream. When changing the dressing, liberal washing of the wound with tepid water is the best and most comfortable way of cleaning the wound.

For small burns, paraffin gauze may be used. For larger wounds, gauze or J-Cloths liberally covered with Flamazine, Betadine or chlorhexidine are better. A layer of wool kept in place by Netelast® or crepe bandage absorbs exudate and supports the burnt area.

Burns of the hands are best treated by putting the hand in a plastic bag (ordinary kitchen ones will do) with a little Flamazine cream. They are lightly bandaged at the wrist over some cotton wool. Much exudate collects, but a daily change and wash is all that is needed. Such treatment allows the mobility of the hand to be preserved and the patient can remain independent since with free hands self-care is possible. When not in use, the hands should be elevated to limit swelling.

Pig skin (fresh or treated by freeze drying) is sometimes applied to the burn wound. It reduces fluid loss and pain and is very good for areas such as the face or chest to which it can be easily applied and changed on alternate

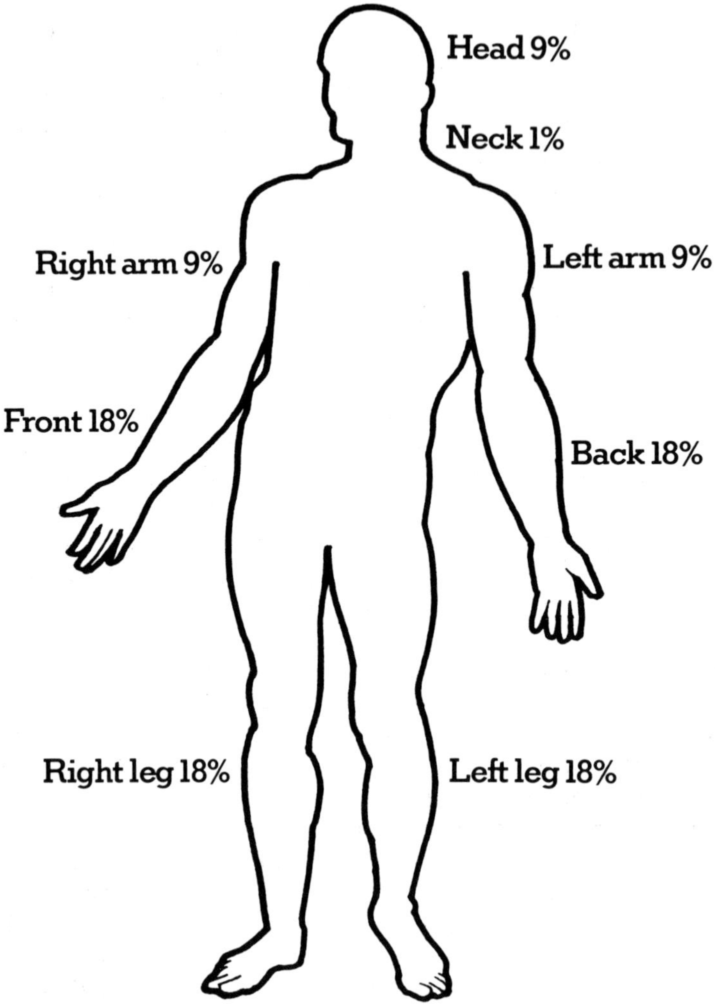

Fig 18.5 'Rule of nine' for calculating the percentage of the body burned.

days. It is very difficult to apply around the mouth, eyes or on the hands.

Early surgery to excise dead skin and to graft the defect should be considered since the risk of infection is reduced and healing may be accelerated. Small, deep wounds may be excised and grafted immediately. This is imperative if an important structure (tendon or joint) is under a deep burn. Larger, full thickness burns, involving less than 10% of the surface are usually excised and grafted before the 5th day (Fig 18.5). Occasionally part of a much more extensive burn is operated upon as soon

as the shock phase (first 48 hours) is over.

Surgery requires special skill and is time-consuming. Inevitably almost every major burn will come to surgery at some stage. The decision as to what operation to do, and when, is based on the combined judgement of the nursing and medical team, so that the best quality of early healing, in the light of the general state of the patient, can be achieved. Surgery for burns patients requires skilled anaesthesia, and there may be anaesthetic problems even with minor burns. The operation is in two stages; the first is excision or desloughing in which the dead tissues are excised or avulsed. If possible, this is performed under tourniquet to reduce bleeding. A clean, dry bed is a good surface for the second stage, a skin graft. Sometimes grafting is delayed if the wound is not clean or dry. There is then a choice of which graft to use.

Small areas covering critical tissues, for example, the palm of the hand, can be resurfaced using full thickness skin in the form of free grafts or flaps. Larger areas can be covered, as a temporary measure, with freeze-dried lyophilised pig skin but it is only a dressing. It can be applied to excised wounds or granulating surfaces to prepare them for autografting.

Split skin grafts taken from cadavers are used in some centres. They grow for a short time but, unless tissue typed, have little advantage over pig skin. There is no substitute for split (partial thickness) skin taken from the patient's own unburnt areas. It can either be applied immediately to the burn wound or stored for up to 3 weeks in a refrigerator for later application. The area from which the graft is taken can be allowed to heal and is often 'cropped' again after 10 days. Enough skin of this type is then available (*see* Ch. 19).

When the burns are *very* extensive, only limited donor areas are available from which grafts can be taken. Besides cropping of these areas, meshing is used. The split skin graft is passed through a device which makes short, parallel cuts so that the graft expands into a mesh perhaps six times larger than the original sheet of skin. When laid on the wound, the epidermis spreads in a few days to cover the spaces of the mesh.

Using one of these measures, or a combination of them, infected wounds should be avoided and early healing attained. A granulating wound (a guarantee of a poor scar) should be a thing of the past.

Surgery provides a solution to so many contemporary problems but cannot be applied in all cases. Age, pre-existing disease, fluid or electrolyte imbalance, head, internal or skeletal injury, septicaemia and especially pulmonary problems may prevent operation at the ideal moment from the point of view of the wound. The skill, experience and availability of theatre teams and space may be limited and other patients and conditions may compete for available facilities.

In treating a burn wound the aim remains to make the healing process as comfortable and quick as possible and to produce the best quality scar. At the same time, the general health and morale of the patient must always be considered in the treatment plan. At the end of treatment the patient must have survived, remain well and be able to move his joints through the maximum range of movement the injury allows and have the least possible scarring, not only of the burn wound, but also of the donor sites of the flaps and grafts which have been used in reconstruction.

Burn scars, particularly in coloured skins, have a great liability to thicken and shrink. It has been found that constant pressure on any scar makes it flatter and reduces shrinkage and joint contracture. Carefully tailored elasticated garments should be prepared for any burn scar as soon as healing is complete. Worn continuously for about 6 months the appearance and function of the scar are greatly improved by these garments.

Chapter 19

Aspects of Infection Control and Skin Grafting in Burned Patients

Edward J.L. Lowbury and J.S. Cason*

It is not always realised that a burn or scald is a wound, similar in many ways to other traumatic injuries (e.g. lacerations, or skin 'degloving' of a limb), but with some special complicating factors. Two factors which have particular importance are the presence of necrotic tissue and the greater extent of the injury in burns than that found in other types of wounds. The moist slough and the adjacent damaged and oedematous tissues provide a nutrient medium in which many types of bacteria can grow freely. The more extensive the lesion, the greater the chances of contamination, and small numbers of bacteria, which would be destroyed by the host defences if they settled on living tissue with good blood supply, can multiply in the slough. Losses of protein (including immunoglobulin) and electrolytes, dehydration, anaemia and raised levels of circulating corticosteroids diminish the patient's resistance to infection. It is not surprising that, after the introduction of effective methods of preventing hypovolaemic shock by fluid replacement in the 1940s, infection came to be recognised as the most common cause of death in patients with extensive burns.

INFECTION OF BURNS

Definitions

Unless effective measures are used to prevent contamination of burn wounds, virtually all of them become colonised by bacteria within 12 to 24 hours. The word 'infection' is often used in describing such microbial colonisation, though it usually causes no apparent damage to the wound and the patient. It would be better to reserve the term 'clinical infection' for microbial colonisation causing recognisable pathological effects, e.g. inflammation, suppuration, pyrexia. As infection in burned patients is superimposed on the local and general effects of the burn injury, which include inflammatory and necrotic changes, it is often impossible on inspection to say whether the patient is infected in the way one can when an operation wound suppurates. Septicaemia, marginal cellulitis, hyperpyrexia, and specific lesions — such as the focal haemorrhagic necroses of psuedomonas infection — are clear evidence, but they are rare except in the most extensive burns. Failure of skin grafts occurs in burns colonised by *Streptococcus pyogenes* but may be caused by other factors (e.g. haemorrhage). Labororary investigation for endotoxaemia by the lumulus lysate test, or for neutrophil involvement by the nitroblue tetrazolium (NBT) test, give evidence respectively, of colonisation. Tests showing neutrophil dysfunction indicate a special hazard, but are not in themselves evidence of clinical infection. Nor is the presence of more

* J.S. Cason died during the production of this chapter.

than 10 bacteria per gram of excised tissue, though clearly the denser the bacterial colonisation of slough and the more extensive the burns, the greater is the chance that bacteria will invade healthy tissue adjacent to the slough and, potentially, go on to invade the blood stream.

Burns of superficial partial skin thickness will heal from the surviving germinal layer of epithelium and present no problems of infection. Full skin thickness burns require skin grafting and are at special risk from infection. Deep partial skin thickness burns may be converted to full skin thickness lesions if they are infected.

In addition to the burn wound, the respiratory and urinary tracts of patients with burns may become infected, often with the same bacteria as those which are present on the wounds.

The micro-organism of burn infection

The bacteria that colonise burns include a wide range of organisms present on the skin, in the mouth and in the colon; the same organisms are found in open traumatic wounds and infected surgical wounds. Before the slough separates (usually after 2–3 weeks if it is not excised sooner), there may be an abundance of Gram-negative bacilli including *Pseudomonas aeruginosa*, *Proteus mirabilis*, Klebsiella spp., *Escherichia coli*, Enterobacter spp. and other intestinal coliform bacilli; also *Staphylococcus aureus*, micrococci, diphteroid bacilli, *Streptococcus faecalis* and occasionally *Streptococcus pyogenes* (the haemolytic streptococcus of Group A). After the separation of slough, the Gram-negative bacilli become sparse and the Gram-positive organisms predominate in the exposed granulation tissue. Many other organisms, including clostridia, Bacillus spp., *Bacteroides fragilis* and fungi (especially *Candida albicans*) appear, often for a short period and apparently unable to compete with the staphylococci and Gram-negative bacilli for living space in the burn wound. In most burns there is mixed flora of several different bacterial species.

Of the organisms that colonise burns, *Str.*

pyogenes has a special place. Though today it is usually an irregular and infrequent visitor, and when present very rarely a cause of the invasive fulminant infections for which it was formerly notorious, *Str. pyogenes* differs from all the other bacteria in usually causing the complete failure of skingrafts if present at the time of operation. Its presence, whether or not associated with signs of clinical infection, is therefore always an indication for chemotherapy (*see below*). Of the other bacteria *Ps. aeruginosa* has been a specially important cause of invasive and sometimes fatal infection in patients with severe burns; it can also interfere with skin grafting, though to a much smaller degree than *Str. pyogenes*. The other Gram-negative bacilli, especially Proteus, Providencia and Klebsiella species, can also cause septicaemic invasion. Most burns colonised with these organisms and with *Staph. aureus* show no apparent pathological effects, but outbreaks of infection by epidemic strains of *Staph. aureus* sometimes occur; when this happens in a Burns Unit, staff as well as patients are liable to have boils. Virus infection (especially herpes) and invasive infection by *Candida albicans* have been reported in some centres, but seem to be a rarity in others.

Bacteriological examination of burns

Because it is necessary to treat all burned patients for *Str. pyogenes* infection, regular bacteriological sampling of burns should be regarded as an obligatory component of patient care. A conventional method is to sample at every change of dressings, or daily if the burn is treated by exposure. Cotton wool swabs are used, previously moistened with peptone water or broth-saline and innoculated on standard culture media — blood agar. Examination of culture plates under ultraviolet irradiation makes it possible to recognise *Ps. aeruginosa* after overnight incubation (Fig 19.1). Standard methods are used for identification of the main groups of burn flora and for antibiotic sensitivity.

Information obtained by counts of bacteria in biopsy specimens from burns has been pre-

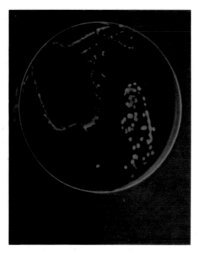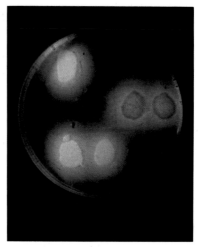

Fig 19.1 Fluorescence under ultraviolet irradiation of *Ps. aeruginosa* growing on blood agar and on a selective medium (cetrimide agar).

ferred by some workers. Biopsy can only be done on very small and possibly unrepresentative portions of the burn, and the laboratory could only undertake a relatively small number of such tests, compared with the numbers of swabs that can be examined. Semiquantitative assessments of swab platings give gradings of density that correlate quite well with biopsy counts from the same burns, provided the samples are taken from burns treated under dressings; the dry eschar of a burn treated by exposure may show relatively few bacteria on its outer surface, though heavily colonised underneath. For this reason quantitative culture from the surface, e.g. on extracts of moistened gauze strips applied to the burn, offers little advantage over semiquantitative swab sampling, for both methods will often underestimate the density of growth in burns treated by exposure method.

Sources and routes of infection

In a Burns Unit most infections with *Ps. aeruginosa* occur by cross-infection from the burns of other patients in the same ward. *Str. pyogenes* and *Staph. aureus* are also acquired in this way and (less often) from respiratory tract carriers of the organisms among members of staff. Self-infection with the flora or skin, mouth and intestinal tract is also common, though the bacteria are often first acquired on these carrier sites from the hospital environment.

Because of their extent and delayed course, burn wounds are more exposed than traumatic or surgical wounds to the hazards of airborne contamination. Staphylococci and other Gram-positive organisms are more likely to be transferred by air than the Gram-negative bacilli, because the latter are much more vulnerable to the lethal effects of desiccation. However, cross-infection with *Ps. aeruginosa* can occur by airborne dispersal from patients during change of dressings though experiments on isolators have shown that *Ps. aeruginosa* is much more likely to be transmitted in the ward by contact than by air. Hands, uniform, contaminated fomites and fluids are potentially important vectors of contact transmission.

A strategy for the prevention of infection in patients with burns, based on knowledge of the sources and routes of transfer, has been developed at the Birmingham Accident Hospital. It envisages the deployment of two 'lines of defence', the first line consisting of measures to prevent contamination of the burn wound, the second line consisting of measures to prevent invasion of the tissues and blood stream by bacteria already colonising the burn (Fig. 19.2).

PREVENTION OF INFECTION

The *first line of defence* has the following components:

1   Primary excision and grafting (suitable only for the smaller full skin thickness burns in which infection would, in any case, be a relatively unimportant problem).
2   Aseptic methods — i.e. physical methods, including sterile handling of wounds by no-touch technique, wearing of protective clothes (especially plastic overalls and gloves for various nursing procedures) and protective isolation techniques.
3   Antiseptic methods — i.e. topical chemoprophylaxis with certain antimicrobal compounds.

The *second line of defence* comprises:

1   Systemic chemotherapy with antibiotics chosen for their activity against bacteria colonising the burns in patients showing clinical signs suggestive of early or impending invasive infection.
2   The use of specific vaccines and immunoglobulins against *Ps. aeruginosa* and, potentially, against other bacteria.
3   General supportive measures, such as control of diabetes, blood transfusion and other measures to restore physiological function.

The following notes summarise ways in which these principles may be applied, with examples drawn from practice at the Burns Unit of the Birmingham Accident Hospital. Since over the years there has been a continuing series of controlled trials of chemotherapy, chemoprophylaxis and other anti-infective measures, no single method can be described as the standard procedure of the Unit; indeed, if any standard exists, it is a state of vigilance for changes in antibiotic sensitivity, necessitating changes in antibiotic regimen. In the earliest controlled trials, a series of patients treated by the untested

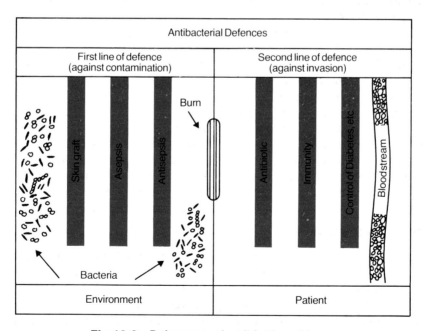

Fig 19.2   Defences against infection of burns.

methods was compared with patients in control series who received no specific therapy or prophylaxis against the relevant organisms; in later trials the unknown method was tested in comparison with control patients who were receiving the current preferred treatments, based on knowledge acquired in previous trials.

First line of defence

Aseptic methods of prophylaxis

1 Use of a plenum ventilated dressing station. One of the methods of reducing contamination by airborne bacteria is the use of a positive pressure-ventilated dressing station. The air, filtered and humidified, is introduced through ceiling inlets to provide 20 air changes per hour; if a 5 minutes' interval is allowed between the departure of one patient and the arrival of the next, the contaminated air is removed and each patient is dressed in air as clean as it was at the beginning of the day.

Indirect evidence of the efficiency of the dressing station was shown by measuring the bacterial content in the air with a silt sampler after dispersal of bacteria from blankets and dressings. Figure 19.3 shows that there was a cumulative increase in contamination of the air when mechanical ventilation was not used, but with mechanical (plenum) ventilation, the level of airborne bacteria fell rapidly from peaks of contamination (B) caused by a sudden dispersal of bacteria. There was heavy contamination of air during the dressing of a large burn, but positive pressure ventilation led to the rapid removal of the cloud of airborne bacteria.

Direct evidence of the value of positive pressure ventilation has been shown by a controlled trial in which one group of patients had burns dressed in the dressing station with the ventilation plant switched on, while the other (control) group was dressed by the same team with the ventilation plant switched off. Figure 19.4 shows that there was a lower incidence of 'hospital' (resistant) *Staph. aureus*, *Str. pyogenes* and *Ps. aeruginosa* on the burn sites dressed with the plenum ventilation switched on.

2 'No-touch' aseptic dressing technique. Prevention of contact transfer involves various procedures, including the 'no-touch' dressing technique, whereby the burned area and dres-

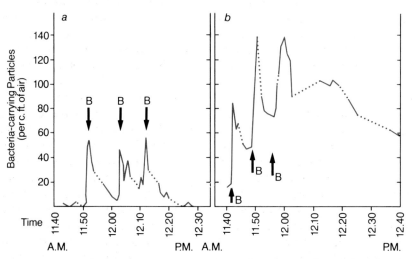

Fig 19.3 Airborne bacterial counts in burn dressing station during dressings with and without plenum ventilation. (From Bourdillon R.B., Colebrook L., 1946. Air hygiene in dressing rooms for burns and major wounds. *Lancet* i: 561, 601).

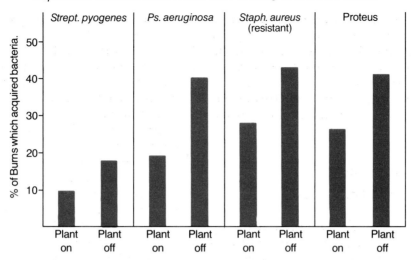

Fig 19.4 Results of controlled trial of plenum ventilated dressing station for burns, showing lower proportions of burns infected with four species of bacteria in patients whose dressings were changed in presence of plenum ventilation (20 air changes/hour).

sings are not touched by human hand. Sterile forceps are used to handle the sterile dressings when they are applied. Disposable sterile surgical gloves can be used for this purpose, provided that care is taken not to touch other objects in the room, and that a fresh pair of gloves is used for each patient.

The dressing team consists of one 'dirty' nurse who removes the old outer dressings and two 'clean' nurses. One of the 'clean' nurses stands behind a trolley which she has prepared, and hands (with sterile forceps) the sterile dressings, kidney dishes, instruments etc. to the second 'clean' nurse, who then dresses the wound.

All nurses and doctors in the dressing station wear caps, masks, gowns and theatre boots or plastic overshoes as in an operating theatre. 'Clean' burns are dressed first; burns infected with *Str. pyogenes* are put at the end of the dressing lists, and burns infected with *Ps. aeruginosa* are placed near the end of the list, but before those infected with *Str. pyogenes* (should such infections be included in the list). When the dressings are finished, the room is thoroughly cleaned and furniture wiped down with a clear soluble phenolic disinfectant. Dirty dressings are put into bins lined with polythene bags, which are then sealed and sent to the incinerator. The patient is covered with freshly laundered sheets and wears a cap throughout the dressing procedure. Bacteriological swabs are taken from the burn sites for subsequent examination in the laboratory as described above.

3 Isolation and isolators. Barrier nursing in an open ward may have some value in preventing transfer of infection by contact, but it has no effect on airborne transfer of bacteria. The conversion of an open 'Nightingale' ward into one with 2-bed and single-bed cubicles in the Birmingham Burns Unit did not lead to any reduction in the incidence of streptococcal, staphylococcal or pseudomonas infection; when half of the cubicles were provided with air conditioners giving 10 air changes per hour of filtered, partially recirculated air, airborne staphylococcal counts were halved, but there was no fall in the burn infection rate. A plastic ventilated isolator (Fig 19.5) was found to cause a significant reduction in *Ps. aeruginosa* infection, but the effects on other bacteria were negligible because an isolator could not prevent self-infection with intestinal, oral or skin organisms, and the isolation system was im-

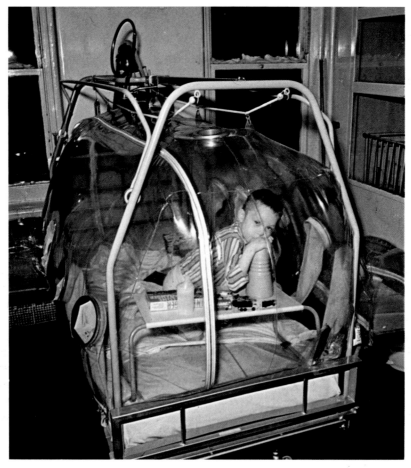

Fig 19.5   A plastic ventilated isolator for protective isolation of burn patients showing glove ports for handling patient and service pouches.

perfect (e.g. food was not sterilised). Plastic isolators are difficult to use, especially in patients with extensive burns; the larger the area of the burn and the more helpless the patient, the more difficult are the nursing problems.

Antiseptic methods of prophylaxis

The application of a topical antimicrobial compound in a cream or lotion is another component of the first line of defence, and one shown by controlled trials to be particularly effective.

Many agents have been used and controlled clinical trials have been done on some of them. The purpose is to prevent cross-infection or 'self-infection'. Most fresh burns and scalds are sterile in the first few hours from the time

of burn injury. If the burn could be completely sealed off from its surroundings by sterile dressings, theoretically it should be possible to prevent cross-infection, particularly if, at the same time, another barrier in the form of an antiseptic or antibiotic application is used in the dressing. This is the principle of the 'closed' method of the treatment of burns with dressings. Although this has been more successful in the treatment of small rather than extensive burns, controlled trials have shown that bacterial colonisation, pyrexia and mortality are reduced in extensive burns by some form of topical chemoprophylaxis. It is customary not to rely on one method for the antimicrobial protection of an extensive burn;

other barriers (e.g. systemic antibiotics, isolators and immunoprophylaxis) can contribute to the protection of the burned patient and help to prevent invasion of the blood stream by bacteria from the infected burn. Routine chemoprophylaxis with broad-spectrum antibiotics, however, must be avoided because of the likelihood of emergence of resistant strains and of opportunist pathogens, with a consequent loss of prophylactic or therapeutic usefulness of these agents. Most locally applied agents have both advantages and disadvantages, and no single agent is ideal.

Silver nitrate (0.5%) compresses. When applied daily and kept moist, compresses of 0.5% silver nitrate have been found to be effective in preventing the growth of *Ps. aeruginosa* on extensive fresh burns (Fig 19.6). However, they have no therapeutic effect, i.e. they do not remove *Ps. aeruginosa* from a burn already colonised by that organism. The application of such a hypotonic solution is likely to cause hyponatraemia, hypokalaemia and hypocalcaemia, so that extra supplements of salt and potassium have to be given, and

frequent serum and urine elecrolyte investigations are necessary; methaemoglobulinaemia is another (infrequent) side effect. The continually wet dressings (day and night) of silver nitrate solution make the patient uncomfortable and cause the staining of the bedclothes. Alternative methods of topical chemoprophylaxis are therefore desirable.

Mafenide. Mafenide acetate (11%) in a cream has been found useful as a prophylactic application and may also have some value in therapy of established pseudomonas infections. Unfortunately, it is a painful form of local treatment when used on partial thickness skin loss burns, though it is more tolerable on full thickness burns which are analgesic except at their periphery. It is recommended that mafenide acetate cream should be 'buttered' with a gloved hand on the surface of the burn, which is then left exposed. Metabolic acidosis may occur when mafenide is applied to extensive burns, but is reversible on stopping the treatment. In a controlled trial mafenide cream was as effective as 0.5% silver nitrate compresses in controlling infection

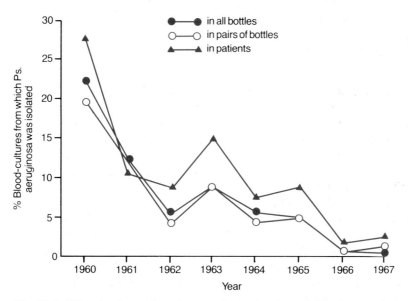

Fig 19.6 Blood cultures from burn patients showing a fall in the proportion of cultures yielding *Ps. aeruginosa* to negligible levels after the introduction of 0.5% silver nitrate compresses in 1965.

with pseudomonas, but less effective against some other bacteria.

Silver sulphadiazine (1%) cream This is the most popular prophylactic application at the present time, and it is useful in prophylaxis against *Ps. aeruginosa* and some other infections. In a controlled trial on extensively burned patients, it was found to compare favourably with silver nitrate compresses as a prophylactic application, with much greater activity against miscellaneous Gram-negative bacilli (coliforms), though slightly less active against *Ps. aeruginosa*. A potential disadvantage was the emergence of a high incidence of sulphonamide-resistant Enterobacteria, including Klebsiella spp., associated with a plasmid which determined the transfer of resistance to sulphonamides and also to several antibiotics.

Silver nitrate-chlorhexidine cream. This cream, containing 0.5% silver nitrate and 0.3% chlorhexidine gluconate, is a useful prophylactic agent, well tolerated and comparable in effectiveness with silver sulphadiazine cream, though less stable. It is an appropriate alternative to silver sulphadiazine cream when sulphonaminde-resistant strains of Gram-negative bacilli have become common in a burns ward. In a controlled trial it was found to be approximately as effective as silver sulphadiazine in excluding *Staph. aureus*, *Ps. aeruginosa*, Proteus spp. and coliform bacillí from burns. A tulle gras dressing containing chlorhexidine has been shown to have prophylactic value against *Staph. aureus*.

Cerium (cerous) nitrate cream. Recently, cerous nitrate applications have been advocated as effective agents for topical chemoprophylaxis. A controlled trial in Birmingham has shown a cerous nitrate cream to have less prophylactic action than silver nitrate-chlorhexidine cream.

Second line of defence

Chemotherapy
Systemic chemotherapy has two prophylactic roles:

1 The removal of reservoirs of infection, as when a *Str. pyogenes* infection is successfully treated.
2 Early treatment of a severe local infection, to prevent invasion when this seems a likely development.

Routine chemoprophylaxis by broad-spectrum antibiotics is an undesirable practice, and likely to fail through the selective encouragement of resistant bacteria; if these proceed to cause septicaemia or other clinical infections, there may be no effective antibiotic available for much needed therapeutic use.

Active and passive immunisation
Promising results of immunoprophylaxis by *Ps. aeruginosa* vaccines and antisera have been reported. An improved polyvalent *Ps. aeruginosa* vaccine, developed at the Birmingham Accident Hospital, has been further developed at the Wellcome Research Laboratories. Trials in normal human volunteers and in burns patients have given very promising results and a pilot controlled trial in India, which is still in progress, has shown the new vaccine to have life-saving potential (Table 1). The vaccine appears to have cross-protective properties

Table 1
MORTALITY OF PATIENTS IN CONTROLLED TRIALS OF PSEUDOMONAS VACCINE

Treatment group	Mean age (yr)	No. of deaths
Vaccinated	1.5–9	0/9
	19 –45	0/9
Unvaccinated	1 –9	3/10
	17 –46	5/10

With acknowledgements to Drs R.J. Jones, E. Roe and J.L. Gupta

against some other Gram-negative bacilli. A specific antipseudomonas immunoglobulin prepared from the plasma of vaccinated volunteers has been found to enhance the immunological protection of severely burned patients, especially if treatment is delayed.

TREATMENT

General

The only organism for which chemotherapy is always indicated when it appears in a burn is the haemolytic streptococcus of Group A (*Str. pyogenes*). This bacterium will usually cause the complete failure of skin grafts, but can almost always be removed within 3 or 4 days by a course of oral treatment with flucloxacillin or cloxacillin, or with erythromycin; systemic penicillin G commonly fails to remove the streptococcus from the burn wound because of the inactivating effect of penicillinase produced by other bacteria in the same burn.

When there are clinical signs of sepsis or septicaemic invasion by other bacteria (e.g. *Staph. aureus*, *Ps. aeruginosa*, *Klebsiella aerogenes*), a course of an antibiotic or antibiotics shown by sensitivity tests to be active against the organisms should be given at full dosage. Clinical criteria are required to judge whether chemotherapy is needed; the most important criterion — and the most dangerous infective complication — is septicaemia, the diagnosis of which is based on a combination of clinical signs and positive blood culture.

Septicaemia

Septicaemia may occur at any time after the admission of a patient and is most likely to occur in the most extensively burned patients though, occasionally, even a small burn may be the source of such an invasive infection. The organism involved is usually one (and sometimes more than one) of the pathogenic microbes which colonise the burned area. Common types include *Staph. aureus*, *Ps. aeruginosa*, *E. coli* or other Gram-negative bacilli, and occasionally fungi (e.g. *Candida albicans*); *Ps. aeruginosa* has been a particularly important and commonly fatal invader. Septicaemia has been said to account for over 50% of deaths in extensive burns, but it is often combined with other debilitating or fatal complications, such as anaemia, bronchopneumonia, hypovolaemia and renal failure.

Any patient with a continuously high temperature (over 103°F), particularly if mental confusion is present, should be suspected of having septicaemia; hallucinations may occur in such patients. Frequent blood cultures should be taken to identify the responsible organisms and their sensitivity to the various antibiotics; it is important that blood culture should be obtained before chemotherapy is started. Some severely burned patients with pseudomonas septicaemia develop leucopenia and hypothermia, and occasionally there appear, on the burns and on normal skin, focal haemorrhagic necrotic lesions which may develop into ecthymatous ulcers. Biliverdinuria has also been found in such patients. Terminal and late signs of invasive infection include paralytic ileus, jaundice, oliguria, endotoxic shock and degeneration and atrophy of previous healthy granulations which become pale and unhealthy in appearance with necrotic areas. Petechial haemorrhages and a palpably enlarged spleen, which are often described in medical cases of septicaemia, are rare in patients with septicaemia complicating burns.

If treatment is to succeed, it is often necessary to make a diagnosis before blood culture results are reported. Sometimes, where antibiotic therapy has already been started, or for reasons unknown, the blood culture of patients with clinical signs of septicaemia may be negative. When no bacteriological findings of burn culture are available in such patients, the treatment must of necessity be blind, and a broad-spectrum bactericidal antibiotic such as gentamicin (or, if gentamicin-resistant strains are prevalent, amikacin) must be used on suspicion of septicaemia. Where previous bacteriological reports on the burn site are available, the predominant organisms found there may be thought to be the cause of the septicaemic state and, while culture reports are awaited, antibiotics active against these bacteria are prescribed. Blind treatment with antibiotics should be avoided whenever possible, because of the risk of choosing one to which the organism is insensitive. The patient receiving such treatment should be isolated, to reduce the likelihood of transmitting resistant variants (should they emerge) to other patients.

Supportive therapy for septicaemic patients include high protein, high calorie diet, repeated blood transfusion to correct anaemia and hypovolaemia, antipyretics, and correction of fluid and electrolyte imbalance. If the 'sick cell syndrome' occurs, it may be treated with glucose, insulin and intravenous therapy. Other supportive treatment includes topical chemotherapy with appropriate antiseptic, antibiotic or antifungal agents and, if necessary, e.g. in gas gangrene (a very rare complication) surgical excision of affected areas. Treatment with hyperbaric oxygen and very large doses of penicillin are also indicated in gas gangrene.

The intravenous route is recommended for systemic chemotherapy of septicaemia, when this is possible, and a higher dosage than the usual dose is required; 'desperate conditions require desperate measures'. Blood levels of the antibiotic may have to be measured to determine the most effective dose; this is particularly important when there is renal failure,

and the optimum length of extended intervals between doses of gentamicin or other aminoglycosides can be judged from results of such assays.

The sodium-potassium ratio of the urine may be reversed in the case of septicaemia, but this may also occur in other 'stress' conditions, such as hypovolaemia and anaemia. Nevertheless, it can be used as corroborative evidence of septicaemia when other signs, such as high temperature and mental confusion, are present.

Skin grafting

Methods

One of the greatest advances in the treatment of extensive burns since the Second World War has been the development of skin grafting (Fig 19.7), due mainly to expansion of the plastic surgery services and training of surgeons in the art of grafting.

Once the burn wound has been successfully closed and treated by means of skin graft, bacteria, which were present on the burn before grafting, rapidly disappear — if they have not themselves caused the destruction of

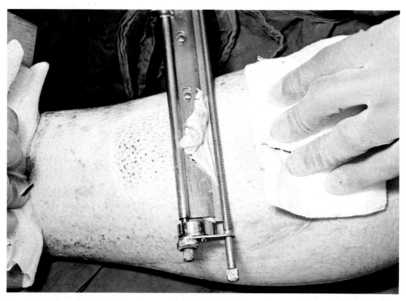

Fig 19.7 Split thickness graft taken with modified Humby knife.

the skin graft. Small full thickness skin loss burns are easily repaired soon after the injury by means of skin grafts, but for the extensive burns grafting is difficult and can often not be performed until the slough has separated by proteolytic digestion (i.e. after 3 weeks or more). It is preferable to close the wound by means of autografts (Figs 19.8; 19.9; 19.10; 19.11) but where the donor sites for these are limited, homografts may also be used with advantage and various techniques have been devised to enhance their effectiveness. One such technique is the 'mesh autograft' (Fig 19.12) covered with homografts when autografts are in short supply and another is the ½″ alternative homograft and autograft strip method (Fig 19.13).

The strips of exposed tissue on rejection of homograft strips, and the spaces of the mesh graft, are bridged by lateral migration from the autograft epithelium. The homografts can be taken from donors or, preferably, from recently deceased persons (cadavergrafts). These have been found to be viable for over a

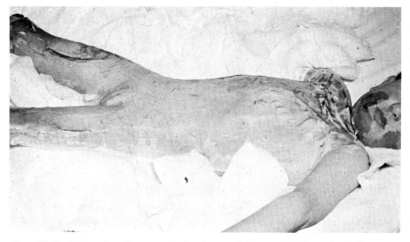

Fig 19.8 Extensive burn sustained on clothes catching alight from unguarded fire, on day 1.

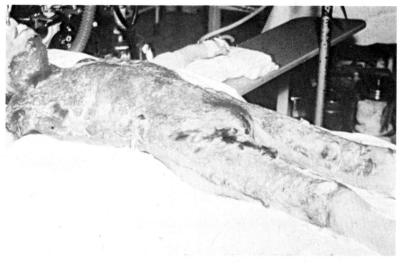

Fig 19.9 Appearance at 3 weeks from the time of burn; now ready for skin grafting.

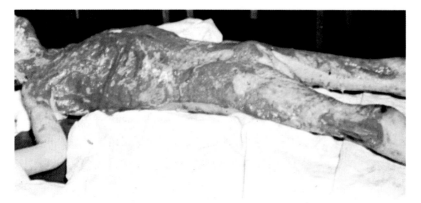

Fig 19.10 After removal of residual sloughs and cleaning of granulations with dry gauze.

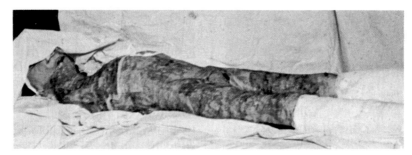

Fig 19.11 Appearance after autografts applied on tulle gras.

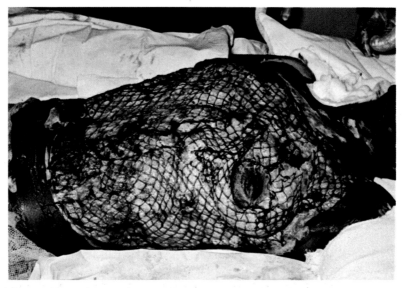

Fig 19.12 Appearance of mesh graft after application to excised full thickness burn of trunk.

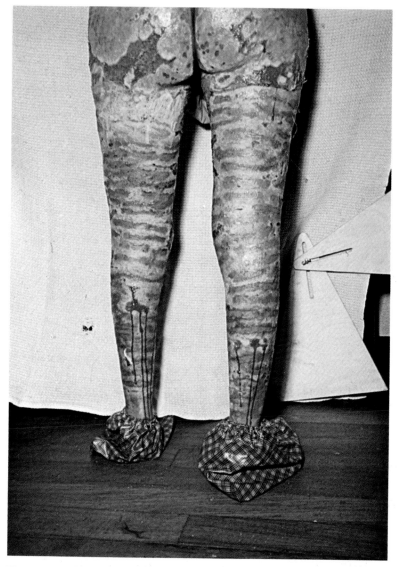

Fig 19.13 Appearance of alternate ½″ strips of autograft and homograft.

year when stored in liquid nitrogen in a vacuum flask. Other substitutes for autografts are less effective; e.g. freeze dried porcine skin xenografts, (Fig 19.14) are rejected more rapidly than homografts. They may, however, have a place where homografts are not available. On rare occasions, when the patient is desperately ill from infection and not fit for anaesthetic or operation, but when the burn is suitable for grafting, it is appropriate to cover the whole of the granulations with homografts as a dressing. If the homograft 'takes', infection may completely disappear, and a child who had been desperately ill, with a high swinging temperature, will then become fit and apyrexial within a few days.

One of the difficulties with skin grafting is diagnosis of the depth of the burn — i.e. whether it has destroyed the full thickness of the skin or has caused only partial skin thick-

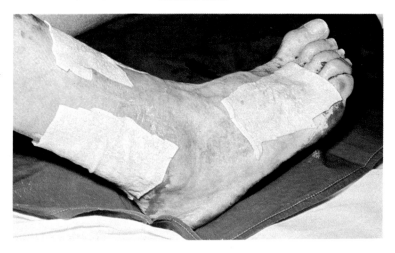

Fig 19.14　Appearance of freeze-dried porcine skin applied to burn (xeno-graft).

ness destruction. For full thickness skin loss burns, early excision of dead tissue and skin grafting is the ideal treatment when this is possible, but if diagnosis of depth of burning is in doubt, a waiting period of some 3 weeks may be necessary before the depth of burn declares itself. It is during this 3 weeks' waiting period before grafting that the patient is in special hazard from invasive and potentially fatal infection. Supportive treatment during this time is given in the form of blood transfusions to correct the anaemia, systemic antibiotics for clinical infection, if present, and high-protein, high calorie diet to correct protein losses associated with the raised metabolic rate.

The technique of tangenital excision (Figs 19.15; 19.16; 19.17) whereby thin slices of the deep partial skin loss burn are removed down to viable tissue and then grafted is another useful method for burns in which there is a mixture of full skin thickness and deep partial skin thickness destruction. The full thickness part of the burn can be excised in the usual

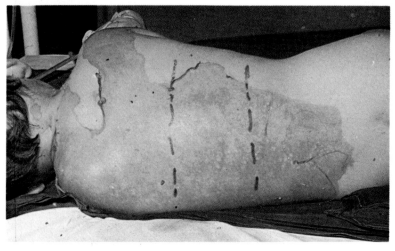

Fig 19.15　Appearance of deep partial (or deep dermal) burn of back. Insensitive to 'pin-prick' text.

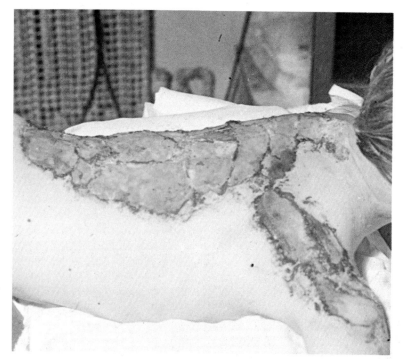

Fig 19.16 Appearance of same burn 4 days after tangential excision and grafting.

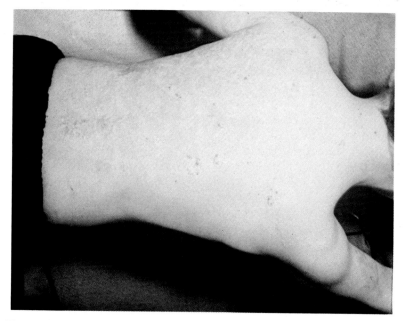

Fig 19.17 Appearance of same burn 18 months after tangential excision. Note absence of hypertrophic scarring.

way with a scalpel, and the deep partial thickness part of the burn can be removed by the tangenital excision. In addition to reducing infection by shortening the time to closure of the wound, it has been claimed that tangenital excision reduced the amount of scarring.

Graft failure

The presence of bacteria other than *Str. pyogenes* on the surface of the burn is not a contraindication to skin grafting. *Str. pyogenes* is an absolute contradindication and should first be removed by means of a systemic course of erythromycin or of a penicillinase-stable penicillin (e.g. flucloxacillin); graft failure is almost inevitable if the streptococcus is not removed, but this can almost always be achieved in 3 to 4 days. Other bacteria, such as *Staph. aureus*, streptococci of other groups, *Ps. aeuruginosa*, Klebsiella spp., Proteus spp., etc., usually do not cause extensive or total failure of skin grafts, and though some of them, especially *Ps. aeruginosa*, may often cause partial failure of skin grafts, it is unjustifiable to delay grafting until the organisms are removed; not only are the bacteria less damaging than *Str. pyogenes* to the grafted skin, but it is much less certain that they will be removed by a course of chemotherapy even when they are sensitive to the antibiotic chosen by *in vitro* tests. In the tangenital excision method of skin grafting, there is always a small amount of microscopic necrotic dermis left, and it would appear that the *Ps. aeruginosa* thrives in this environment and can destroy the graft. Other causes of skin graft failure include inadequate haemostasis, with haematoma formation under the graft, and also insufficient fixation of the graft ('slipping'), so that the newly formed connecting capillaries from grafted site to graft are destroyed, leading to loss of circulation in the graft.

Contractures, scarring and deformity

An extensive burn may require several thin split thickness skin grafting operations before the wound is finally closed and infection removed, and the patient may be in hospital for as long as 3 months or more. Even when the burn is finally healed, other complications, such as deep vein thrombosis and pulmonary embolus, may occur and the deformities and disabilities due to contracture of the scarring may involve the postconvalescent patient in many plastic surgical and skin grafting operations for several years afterwards. Contractures of the face, including ecropion of eyelids, may involve repeated operations for reconstruction of nose, ears, etc (Fig 19.18). Likewise, deformities of the hands may require many corrective full thickness (Wolfe) grafts on the flexor aspects of the fingers and the cleft between thumb and index finger, and arthrodesis of joints in optimum position for best function. These operations are tedious for the patient and, even after many operations, there may still be obvious scarring and unsatisfactory cosmetic results, though function can usually be improved.

To help those patients who still suffer from cosmetic defects of the face, head and hands (the parts of the body which cannot be covered by clothing), there are various methods of skin camouflage. These include wigs where baldness with scarring has occurred, various prostheses, including artificial noses and eyes attached to spectacles, artificial plastic ears which can be fixed to the side of the head and artificial limbs. A new speciality of consultant camouflage experts has evolved, advising patients as to the various cosmetic creams, powders and other preparations which can help; they also advise as to the best way of covering scars, marks and blemishes, as well as the best types of cosmetics to use.

Tube pedicles, flaps and 'z'-plasties can be used to repair various contractures, particularly about the neck, and more recently 'free' flaps have been used whereby the portion of the skin and fat receives a blood supply by direct microsuture of arteries and veins of the flap to corresponding vessels at the site of repair (e.g. neck and leg).

The shock room

At the Birmingham Accident Hospital all pa-

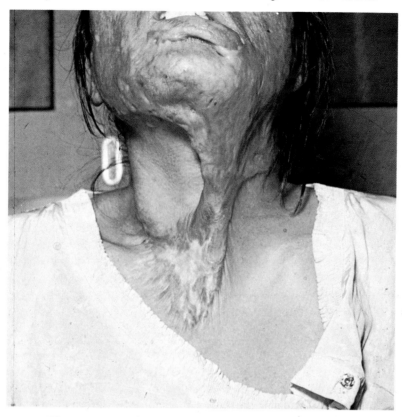

Fig 19.18 Appearance of contracture of left side of neck.

tients with burned areas greater than 10% (in children) or 15% (in adults) of the body surface, excluding erythema, are admitted to a special shock room for intensive care. This is provided with facilities for intravenous transfusion, oxygen and suction supplies; mechanical ventilation with clean filtered air is desirable in the shock room. Special nurses are in attendance for the whole of the shock treatment (48 hours); they wear caps, masks, gowns and plastic overshoes or theatre boots, and use aseptic techniques described above in handling and dressing the patient. The room and furniture are cleaned before admission of a new patient with a clear soluble phenolic disinfectant correctly diluted to the manufacturer's recommendations. A urinary catheter is passed, and the nurse measures the volume of urine passed hourly; she is also responsible for the control of the rate of intravenous infusion ordered by the doctor, and keeps an intake and output fluid balance chart.

The preferred colloid intravenous transfusion fluids for prevention or treatment of hypovolaemic shock are human plasma or plasma protein fraction and/or Dextran '110'. The usual methods of assessing the volume of colloid to be transfused include standard formulae, urine output, haematocrit measurements and classical signs and symptoms of shock (blood pressure, pulse etc.). A formula in common use for adult patients is 1–1.5 litres of plasma for every 10% of the body surface burned in the first 24 hours, half of this being given in the first 8 hours and the other half in the next 16 hours. If the patient is a child, the formula is one plasma volume for every 15% of the body surface burned. In the second 24-hour period about half these amounts are required.

All persons entering the shock room wear caps, masks, gowns and 'bootees' or overshoes, as in an operating theatre; they wash their hands with a chlorhexidine gluconate detergent formulation or rub with an alcoholic lotion on arrival and before leaving.

Intake of oral fluids by the patient is restricted to 75% of the normal intake per hour and should be in the form of an isotonic saline bicarbonate solution; water may cause 'water intoxication' or encephalopathy in children.

Intravenous infusion bottles should be changed every 4 hours because the colloid may act as a culture medium for any accidental contamination by bacteria, leading to heavy colonisation in a few hours. This is a particularly important precaution when only small volumes of plasma (e.g. 50ml/h) are being given, as in the treatment of infants, and should be observed even if it means wasting some of the contents of the bottle.

Great aseptic care should be taken in setting up an intravenous infusion or transfusion, and the area of skin should be thoroughly disinfected before use (e.g. with 70% ethanolic solution containing 0.5% chlorhexidine, applied with friction). Prolonged central vein catheterisation should be avoided if at all possible. All intravenous catheters should be removed as soon as possible after the completion of shock treatment to minimise the risk of infection.

The temperature of the room should be in the region of 80–90°F to avoid shivering with consequent hyperpyrexia and raised metabolism.

Ward procedures

Nurses attending extensively burned patients wear masks and plastic aprons or gowns. They wash hands with an antiseptic detergent and water or, preferably, rub to dryness with 70% ethanol or isopropanol before and after attending to the patient; if alcohol is applied, the solution should contain 1% glycerol or another suitable emollient to prevent excessive drying of the skin. The use of disposable sterile gloves is an added precaution, but care should be taken that other objects in the cubicle are not touched before handling the patient. Patients with *Str. pyogenes* infection should be placed in source isolation, preferably in single-bed cubicles. Patients requiring isolation for other reasons include those being treated with the reserve antibiotics, such as amikacin or fusidic acid, in order to prevent cross-infection should resistant variants emerge. Patients with infectious diseases such as measles, food poisoning and chicken pox should, if the burns are too extensive for transfer to an isolation hospital, also be isolated in the Burns ward. During an outbreak, admissions may have to be limited to children already immunised against the epidemic organism, and if the epidemic is large, closure of the ward or wards may become mandatory. Reopening should be preceded by a complete and thorough cleaning of the ward furniture, floors, walls, etc. For prevention of some infections, uninfected children may have to be treated with gamma globulin or a specific immunoglobulin.

Doctors examining patients should take care to wash hands (preferably applying alcohol or alcoholic chlorehexidine and rubbing to dryness) before and after contact with the patient. Subdivision of the wards into cubicles will not necessarily prevent cross-infection; though mechanical ventilation of cubicles with filtered air was found to reduce the numbers of airborne staphylococci, it did not reduce the incidence of staphylococcal infection, and even isolators (*see above*) had only a limited effect and against only one of the bacteria studied.

However, isolation of extensively burned patients in a Burns Unit — and source isolation of any burned patient in a general surgical ward — is desirable (in the Burns Unit for convenience of nursing). Cubicle isolation has the advantage of making it possible to have mixed male and female wards, thus helping to use beds more efficiently. In a Burns Unit disposable bed pans are not recommended because pieces of dressing material are likely to be deposited in the pans with the excreta, and these can clog the effluent from the bed pan disintegrators. A bed pan washer-disinfector should be used for non-disposable bed pans.

Physiotherapy

Active physiotherapeutic methods are essential for the well-being of the extensively burnt patient. To prevent pressure sores the patient should be moved into a different position every 2 hours by day and by night, either manually or by means of special mechanical beds and mattresses. The risk of respiratory complications can be reduced by breathing exercises, postural drainage, 'clapping', and 'sucking and bagging' where necessary. Early mobilisation of all parts of the body, when this is possible, may prevent stiffness, and is particularly important in burns of the hand. Active hand exercises should be started immediately in the case of partial skin loss burns and the 'hand bag' treatment, using a polythene bag with an antimicrobal cream inside, is an ideal method. In some full skin thickness burns of the hand, it may be necessary to wait until the burn is healed by skin grafting before exercises can be started.

Prevention of contractures requires the use of suitable splintage of the affected parts for a few weeks, but success is not always achieved, as there is a limit to the permissible duration of splintage because of the danger of stiffness occuring in the joints with prolonged immobilisation.

Immersion of the burns in a Hubbard tank or bath is practised in some Burns Units as part of the early local treatment of the burned patient to facilitate separation of slough. In Birmingham, it has been preferred to use the baths in the late stages of treatment when the wound is virtually healed; it is then mainly of use for exercise of weak or stiff limbs, and also for removal of debris and to improve the patient's sense of well-being. It is a sensible precaution to use a disposable polythene liner of the bath for each patient, as well as giving the bath a thorough cleansing and disinfection with a clear soluble phenolic disinfectant after use in order to reduce the chances of cross-infection.

The physiotherapist should take full precautions against cross-infection, and should wash her hands (preferably with 70–95% alcohol or alcoholic 0.5% chlorhexidine) before and after handling the patient; she should wear disposable sterile gloves while handling patients with unhealed burns.

Chapter 20

Some Medico-Legal Aspects of Wounds

A. Keith Mant

The recognition of the type of wound or wounds and the examination of their distribution may enable the wound or wounds to be classified immediately as likely to be accidental, suicidal or homicidal. Overlap of their designation not infrequently occurs, but an understanding of wounding may enable a doctor who is confronted by an injured patient to assess with reasonable accuracy whether the injuries are the result of a criminal assault. If so, the sooner the police are notified, the more probable will be the apprehension of the assailant.

In common with all medical or surgical investigations, a full history of how the injury occurred is important. Such a history may upon occasions have a profound influence upon the final assessment of the case. If the patient is unconscious when seen, one must make use of the history supplied by those who saw the incident or conveyed the patient to hospital. In cases of an alleged criminal assault, the doctor carrying out the examination of the injured person must be able to satisfy himself whether the injuries are consistent or not with the story he has been given. He will probably have to give this opinion later in court and be cross-examined upon how he arrived at his conclusions should someone be charged with an offence. A good history is particularly important when a patient complains that he or she has been assaulted, especially in cases of alleged sexual

assaults. In some cases the nature, pattern and distribution of the injuries is such that they bear no resemblance to the assault alleged by the patient.

Wounds are divided into three types and it is important that these three types of wound should be recognised. Overlap occurs which may make recognition difficult.

BLUNT IMPACT INJURIES

In a forensic connotation, blunt impact injuries often conjure up lurid visions of assailants battering their victims senseless with an assortment of club or club-like weapons. In practice, this is unusual. Most blunt impact injuries are accidental. In everyday practice the least serious of these injuries generally result from falls and the more serious from road traffic accidents.

Blunt impact injuries are divided into three groups.

Abrasions

Abrasions are mere scratches of the skin and are caused by movement between the blunt object and the skin. The movement may be mainly sideways producing a 'scraping abrasion' (Fig 20.1) or inwards causing a 'pressure abrasion'.

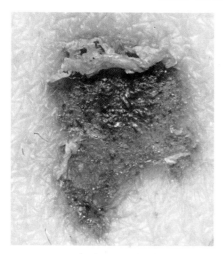

Fig 20.1 Scraping abrasions. The heaping up of the epidermis is well illustrated.

Abrasions are important in forensic practice because they may:

1 mark the point of contact between the blunt instrument and the patient;
2 reproduce a mirror image of the shape of the leading edge of the blunt instrument;
3 be the only external indication of a deep injury.

In the living, abrasions may scab over and eventually heal without scarring. Abrasions which are perimortal, or even postmortem, dry and often have a yellow parchment-like colour and are depressed below the general skin surface. The superficial excoriation of the skin which is sometimes seen in the napkin area of infants who are unwell, dries in a similar manner. The resultant depressed dried areas may suggest a serious lack of care to those who do not recognise them for what they are.

Contusions or bruises

Contusions or bruises occur as a result of the rupture of subcutaneous or deeper blood vessels following an impact (Fig 20.2). The skin may be intact, abraded or lacerated (*see below*). Bruises spread, occupying a greater area than the leading edge of the instrument which

caused them. Deep bruises may take several days before they have spread sufficiently to become visible to the naked eye and may only become visible some distance from the site of impact, having tracked along the tissue planes. Bruises develop most readily in lax tissues such as around the eye (black eye). They are frequently surmounted by an abrasion marking the point of impact if this occurs over a bony area. When a bruise has formed, the fluid element of the blood is absorbed back into the blood stream. If the deep bruising is extensive, as may occur following judicial or other beatings with heavy canes, death may occur several days later from severe anaemia consequent upon the blood loss into the tissues. The large volume of blood which may be lost from a closed fracture is well recognised by the orthopaedic surgeon. In beating with a light cane or whip, capillaries may rupture in the cutis and the haemorrhage remain localised, thus producing a mirror image of the weapon. Discrete bruising may result from the application of a firm grip. The bruises may be surmounted by finger-nail type abrasions. These gripping injuries are seen on the neck in manual strangulation or throttling and on the arms when persons are forcibly restrained. In cases of child abuse, they may appear on the trunk of the infant. Erythematous wheals, falling short of actual bruising, may be seen after violent slapping. The pattern of the fingers or even the whole hand may be visible

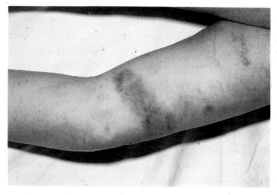

Fig 20.2 Bruising. Linear bruise following impact with a motor vehicle.

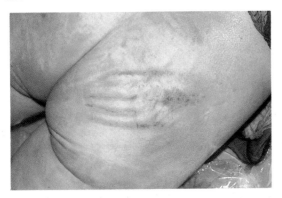

Fig 20.3 A clear handmark upon the buttock of a woman recovered from a stream.

(Fig 20.3). Bruises occur more readily in the very young and the very old. In the very old, they may take some weeks or even months to resolve.

Lacerations

These are splits of the skin caused by crushing of the tissues with blunt impact and occur over the bony prominences which provide the hard surface upon which the skin is crushed. Lacerations must be differentiated from incised wounds. This may be very difficult if the blunt instrument also possesses a cutting edge such as an axe. If the axe is very sharp, it may incise the skin (*see below*) but, if blunt, may primarily crush it. However, as an axe is a heavy weapon, it will inflict much more extensive

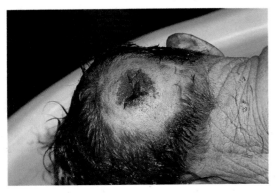

Fig 20.4 A typical laceration following a heavy fall onto the back of the head. Note the irregular tearing of the skin and the surrounding abraded area.

injuries than a knife and even if its cutting edge is very sharp, abrasions will commonly occur along the edges of the skin wound. In lacerations the skin, subcutaneous and deeper tissues are torn apart. Nerve tissue and blood vessels may maintain their continuity and be seen in the depth of the wound. Many lacerations have abraded edges and are usually associated with some degree of bruising. However, as the wound is open, blood will escape through the laceration rather than spread into the soft tissues (Fig 20.4).

From the above description of the three types of blunt impact injury it is apparent that the type of injury produced will not only depend upon the leading edge of the instrument, but also upon the part of the body upon which it impinges itself. To take a simple example, a heavy blow with the clenched fist to the abdomen may cause no injury, the force of the blow being absorbed by the abdominal wall. However, such a blow delivered with identical force to the eye may cause an abrasion, a contusion or even a laceration, or a combination of all three.

INCISED WOUNDS

Whereas blunt impact injuries are usually accidental, incised wounds and penetrating wounds are usually intentional as their character normally implies intent.

Incised wounds are by definition inflicted with a sharp cutting instrument such as a knife (the traditional cut-throat razor is now becoming a rare event). In an incised wound the skin, subcutaneous and deeper tissues are cut through cleanly and any nerve tissue or blood vessels in the path of the instrument will be cut across. Incised wounds are usually self-inflicted.

PENETRATING WOUNDS

Penetrating wounds are, in the context of this chapter, wounds in which the depth is greater than the external width and are usually, except in the case of gunshot wounds, inflicted by another person.

Penetrating wounds in this country are usually inflicted with a stabbing instrument such as a dagger (rare), kitchen or carving knives, flick knives or penknives. More rarely, other stabbing instruments such as ice-picks, chisels, screwdrivers, scissors or pokers may be used. The force required to inflict a deep stab wound is very little if the weapon is sharply pointed. After the skin is pierced, there is little resistance to the passage of the instrument unless it strikes bone or its handle comes into contact with the skin. Less commonly in England penetrating injuries are due to firearms or explosives.

It is difficult for a doctor or surgeon to assess the potential danger of a penetrating wound from external examination as the external wound may give no indication of the depth and hence of the damage to vital organs. Even if the stabbing instrument which inflicted the wound is known, it may not be possible to estimate the maximum depth of penetration. In the young, the thoracic cage is compressable and hence a violent stabbed wound may inflict injuries perhaps 2 inches deeper than the length of the blade. Similarly, in cases of abdominal injuries, stabbed wounds with a short blade such as a penknife or paring knife may be at least twice as long as the blade of the instrument. Penetrating injuries due to firearms and explosives are particularly difficult to assess and are especially dangerous in the long term as foreign material may be carried into the wound causing gas gangrene or tetanus.

INTERPRETATION OF WOUNDS

Accidental, suicidal or homicidal

The interpretation of the wounds depends largely upon the pattern of injury. The violence used to inflict the injury may be misleading as, during certain forms of violent self-destruction, the suicide may use incredible force against himself. It may be vital in death following violence of any kind to examine the clothing of the victim in order to arrive at a reasonable reconstruction of how the injuries were inflicted. Thus in all cases of injury all clothing on the patient must be kept, however badly torn or soiled it may be, in case it is required for subsequent expert examination. This applies in all road traffic accidents and especially in 'hit and run' cases.

It is simpler to interpret injuries in general if the patterns of self-inflicted injuries are considered in detail. Any violent death where the injuries do not follow a recognised suicidal patterns must be considered as either accidental or homicidal until proved otherwise.

In considering suicidal injuries the following general characteristics of self-inflicted wounds must be remembered:

1 the site or sites must be accessible to the suicide;
2 suicides do not injure their features;
3 suicides do not as a general rule inflict wounds other than firearm wounds through their clothing;
4 tentative wounds, prior to infliction of the fatal injury, are almost the rule with incised wounds and very common with stab wounds;
5 they are clearly deliberate;
6 they are sometimes inflicted in front of a mirror;
7 they are often centrally placed.

Suicidal blunt impact injuries

These are generally of interest only to the pathologist and coroner and are usually inflicted by jumping off high buildings or in front of trains. Very occasionally, however, self-inflicted injuries are produced by weapons such as hammers or axes. In these rare cases the blows are aimed at the top of the head in the midline and are neatly grouped in this area.

If we consider the following case of homicide we can see how it differs from the general pattern for suicide:

A young woman telephoned the police station to say that her common law husband had committed suicide by striking himself on the head with a hammer which was still held in his hand. When the police arrived the deceased was lying prone. His right arm was beneath his body and the handle of a claw hammer lay in his right hand. The injuries, however, were on the back of the head on the left side and also on the left shoulder. When the scalp was reflected it was quite clear that it would not be possible for such injuries to be self-inflicted on account of their severity, number, position and distribution. Several of the injuries were of such severity that consciousness would almost certainly be lost after any one of them had been inflicted.

The almost mathematical positioning of self-inflicted wounds is illustrated by the following case which, although a head injury, cannot be classified as blunt impact.

The suicide removed the guard from a circular saw and placed his head against it. The saw cut through the skull and the blade passed between the two cerebral hemispheres. The man got up and walked away, finally collapsing from a haemorrhage from the superior sagittal sinus.

Bite marks

Bite marks are a form of patterned blunt impact injury which are seen on children who are the victims of non-accidental injury (battered babies) and victims of sexual assault. It is important that a bite mark should be recognised as it may provide excellent forensic evidence in two ways:

1   a swab taken from a bite mark (or a love bite) may enable the blood group of the

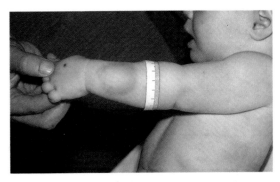

Fig 20.5 A bite mark on the forearm of a nine-month-old infant. The bite was identified as having been inflicted by the father.

assailant to be identified;
2   the pattern of teeth marks may enable the assailant to be identified from his dentition and, most important, will allow many possible suspects to be excluded from the police inquiry.

If a bite mark is suspected, a swab should be taken at once and a forensic odontologist called to examine the injury (Fig 20.5).

Incised wounds

Incised wounds are usually self-inflicted and when they are, they are clearly deliberate. Fatal wounds are usually to the neck, but prior to the infliction of these wounds, tentative cuts are almost invariably present in certain well defined areas. These tentative cuts are most commonly present on the fronts of the wrists, but may also be present on the arms, abdomen or groin. They are parallel to each other or in groups of parallel cuts. The clothing is invariably removed from the area to be assaulted. The number of cuts present depends upon their depth. If they amount to no more than mere abrasions, fifty or more may be present; if they are deep, as few as two or three only may be seen (Fig 20.6).

The tentative cuts may be followed by fatal incised wounds to the throat. The head is thrown back and tentative cuts are found at the beginning of the fatal incision or incisions. The violence used may be incomprehensible to

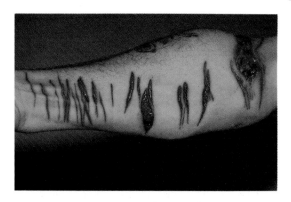

Fig 20.6 Self-inflicted incised wounds of the forearm. These wounds increase in severity as they approach the antecubital fossa where the brachial artery was severed.

those who have never seen self-inflicted neck wounds. The blade usually severs the larynx separating the thyroid and hyoid bones and cuts into or through the anterior longitudinal ligament. Usually, there is more than one such incision. Because the head is thrown back the carotid artery is protected by the transverse processes of the cervical vertebrae. Injury to the carotid arteries suggest homicide. The deliberation of self-inflicted incised wounds is evident from their orderly pattern. It would only be possible to inflict such neck wounds homicidally if the victim were unconscious or held motionless by some other person. Even in such cases the pattern of injury is less orderly than in suicide.

Self-inflicted cuts of a tentative nature are sometimes found upon persons who have committed suicide by some other means, e.g. by poisoning, drowning, etc. The recognition of such self-inflicted wounds is of major importance and may offer a logical explanation in a bizarre case.

Young persons who have emotional or mental problems frequently draw attention to themselves by taking a drug overdose. These gestures or cries for help are well recognised. Less common are those persons who cut themselves and tell the police or the doctor that they have been attacked. These cuts or incised wounds are superficial and, if multiple, run parallel to each other. They may be on the backs of the legs, in which case they usually run parallel with the ground. These wounds must be in areas accessible to the patient and are not found on the face. There are, of course, no defence type wounds. Speedy recognition that these wounds are self-inflicted may save an expensive and prolonged police investigation.

Homicidal incised wounds are unusual in this country and, unless the victim is unconscious or under restraint, show none of the deliberation associated with self-inflicted injuries. A person who is in possession of his or her faculties when attacked will attempt a defence. Wounds may be found through clothing, on parts of the body inaccessible to the deceased and often on the face. Defence wounds (*see below*) are a very common feature of an assault with a cutting instrument. Many incised wounds today are inflicted with broken bottles or glass. Those inflicted by the old fashion 'cut throat razor' are becoming of little more than historical interest.

Stabbed wounds

Stabbed wounds are usually homicidal and may appear anywhere upon the body and not infrequently in areas which preclude self-infliction.

Various types of stabbing instruments have already been listed. The most common stabbing instrument in the domestic scene is a

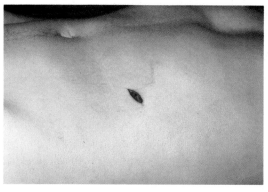

Fig 20.7 The classical appearance of a stabbed wound inflicted with a single-edged knife.

kitchen knife. Examination of the external wound will often give a good indication of the type of instrument used. Kitchen knives are single-edged and injuries caused by single-edged weapons are usually characteristic. The wound will have one clean cut end and one squared or rounded end which may have an abraded edge. (Fig 20.7).

Stabbed wounds inflicted with blunt or relatively blunt leading edges such as a poker will be surrounded by a collar abrasion. Wounds inflicted with a chisel will be rectangular.

Suicidal stabbing does occur and cases vary very little in pattern. The fatal wound is usually through the precordium or, more rarely, below the xiphisternum. Clothing is removed or pulled aside and two or three tentative 'pricks' are usually present in the vicinity of the fatal wound. Occasionally there are several deep wounds.

It is of interest to note that some twenty years ago homicidal stab wounds were almost invariably multiple (Fig 20.8) whereas today single wounds are common. They differ from self-inflicted wounds as they pass through any clothing worn by the deceased over the site of the injury unless the victim is naked. Victims of lethal stabbed wounds may survive for some time without treatment even when the wound involves the heart. Wounds of the right ventricle are more rapidly fatal than those of the left ventricle.

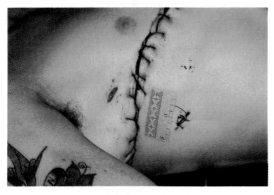

Fig 20.8 The stab wound below the thoracotomy incision has been sutured. The wound above the incision is from a surgical drain.

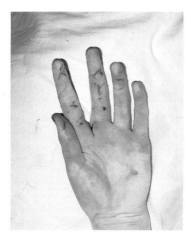

Fig 20.9   Classical defence type injuries of the hand.

Defence wounds

There is one type of wound which should always be looked for in cases of incised or stabbed wounds. These are injuries of a defensive nature.

When anyone who is in possession of their faculties and is unrestrained is attacked with a knife, he or she will endeavour to protect themselves provided they have sufficient warning. They may grab at the knife and receive cuts to the hand (Fig 20.9) or raise an arm and receive stab wounds through the arm. If they are attacked with a blunt instrument, they may place a hand on their head to protect it and have bones of their fingers and hands fractured.

Gunshot wounds

Self-inflicted gunshot wounds merit a section on their own as they are inflicted with such mathematical precision that any deviation from a recognised suicidal site of entry must be considered as accident or homicide unless shown otherwise.

Gunshot wounds are unusual in urban areas and the majority of accidental and suicidal shootings occur in the country. In mainland Britain homicidal shootings and deaths from bomb explosions are still comparatively rare.

In gunshot wounds a bullet or collection of

pellets enter the body at varying velocities depending upon the type of gun and the ammunition. When a gun is discharged, smoke and unburned powder leaves the muzzle of the gun with the projectile. The pressure of the gases behind the projectile may be over 20 tons per square inch.

Guns vary from hand-guns, such as revolvers or automatic pistols firing single projectiles, to long-barrelled guns which must be fired from the shoulder. The latter consist of rifles firing single projectiles and shot guns, which fire a cylinder of pellets that separate soon after leaving the muzzle of the gun.

Self-inflicted wounds to the head are found in certain well defined sites known as the 'sites of election' (Fig 20.10). These sites of election are situated in the centre of the forehead, in the roof of the mouth, behind the symphysis mentis and in either temple, depending upon the right or left handedness of the suicide. One of these sites of election will be chosen even by someone who has never used a gun previously. The author has known cases where a person who has never apparently fired a gun before has bought one and, without any reference to a textbook on forensic medicine, has shot himself correctly through one of the classical 'sites of election'.

For a person to shoot himself the gun must be discharged in close proximity to the skin (excluding the theoretical possibility of an apparatus where the gun is fired from a distance). Usually the muzzle of the gun is pressed against the skin. The resulting wound is a close contact wound. A close contact wound may have a stellate margin due to the gases from the propellant charge expanding beneath the skin and splitting it. Under these circumstances, the entry wound will appear larger than the muzzle diameter of the gun. Powder blackening or tattooing occurs around the entry wound (Fig 20.11; 20.12). The 'sites of election' are the same whether a hand-gun (pistol or revolver), a rifle or a shotgun are

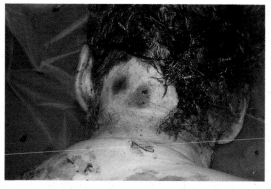

Fig 20.11 Contact homicidal gunshot wounds of the back of the head (.22 rifle).

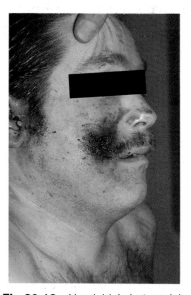

Fig 20.12 Homicidal shotgun injury.

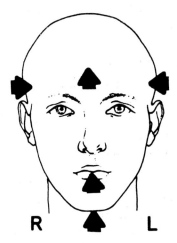

Fig 20.10 Self-inflicted gunshot wounds of the head; the 'sites of election'.

used. When the injury has been inflicted with a hand-gun or rifle an exit wound is not uncommon. Any deviation from a site of election is suspicious and the absence of powder tattooing suggests the gun was not fired by the deceased.

The contact entry wound of a shotgun, except for its size, has all the characteristics of a contact wound inflicted with a hand-gun. When, however, a shotgun is discharged at a distance of 3 feet or more, the shot has already started to separate by the time it reaches the victim and so the entry wound will have first a serrated edge and, at longer distances, separate pellet entry wounds around the principal wound. The exception to this is when the gun is discharged through some resistance, such as a heavy coat, when the shot will begin to spread at once. The smoke from the propellant

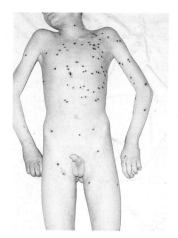

Fig 20.15 Accidental fatal shotgun injury from a distance of approximately 20 yards.

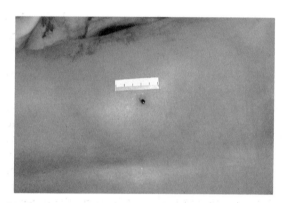

Fig 20.13 Homicidal bullet wound of back, fired from several yards.

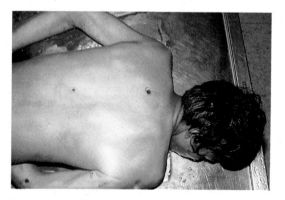

Fig 20.14 Two bullet wounds in the back fired from approximately 20 yards.

gases, however, will still cause powder tattooing around the entry wound.

Self-inflicted firearm wounds of the chest may occur over the front or left side, but do not have such an exact site of election as firearm wounds of the head. A gunshot suicide does not normally bare the chest prior to shooting himself.

All other entry wounds must be considered as accidental or homicidal. Bullet wounds in the back, as in Figs 20.13 and 20.14, are clearly not self-inflicted and likewise the spread of shot in Fig 20.15 indicates that the shotgun was discharged from a distance of some 20 yards.

PROCEDURES THAT SHOULD FOLLOW A VIOLENT DEATH

Whilst the patient is alive every effort is made to resuscitate him, irrespective of any interference with evidence which may aid the police in the reconstruction of the injuries causing death. Once death has occurred, however, nothing should be done to the body. It should not be washed or laid out. Any surgical drains, tracheostomy tubes or intravenous lines should be left *in situ*. Most important, all clothing should be preserved and any blood or urine taken when the patient was admitted should be sealed and retained.

The clothing, blood, urine and other possessions of the deceased will be handed over to the police officer who has the function of 'exhibits officer' in any death due to, or believed to have resulted from, a criminal act. In all other unnatural deaths or deaths reported to the Coroner, the Coroner's Office may take possession of any articles which may be of value to the Coroner's enquiry. This includes any blood or urine collected when the patient was first admitted to hospital.

As soon as a death due to violence or any unnatural cause has occurred, the Coroner should be informed forthwith. The procedure to be followed when a case is reported to the Coroner varies from area to area. In areas where there are regular Coroner's Officers, they will be informed and they, in turn, will inform the Coroner. In other areas reporting is done through the local police station. Whenever a death is referred to the Coroner, the deceased should not be laid out, washed or have medical or sugical apparatus, such as drains or tracheostomy tubes removed without the authority of the Coroner or his pathologist.

The importance of the preservation of such evidence is well illustrated in the following case.

A married couple, who were not on the best of terms, attended a New Year's Eve function at a country club. When the celebrations finished in the early hours of New Year's Day, the husband went to collect his car. He returned with it to the club, but could not locate his wife. She was later found dead in the road. After her death was certified at the local hospital she was moved at once to the mortuary. When she was seen the next day, she had a clear tyre mark in dust across her lower chest and abdomen. The husband, needless to say, was strongly suspected by the police with having been concerned with his wife's death. The tyre pattern, however, upon his wife's body was entirely different from that of his own tyres and so he was at once exonerated. If the lady had been undressed and washed, this

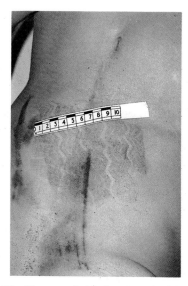

Fig 20.16 Tyre mark in dust on the chest of the deceased.

valuable evidence would have been destroyed and the husband might have been charged with a serious offence (Fig 20.16)

The importance of retaining samples of blood and urine removed from the patient upon admission cannot be over-stressed as they will provide positive evidence of the presence and level of alcohol or drugs in the patient around the time of the incident. When a road traffic accident occurs, for example, there are rarely any eye witnesses. There may be several persons who, on hearing the noise of the impact, will turn around and genuinely believe that they saw the whole incident. For example, a drunken pedestrian may stagger off the footpath in front of a motor vehicle. The 'eye witness' account may suggest that the driver of the car was to blame for the accident and not the pedestrian. If the injured patient survives for a day or longer in hospital and the original samples of blood and urine have not been kept, there may be no evidence to show that the deceased was inebriated at the time of the accident. It is not rare to find blood alcohols of 300–400 mg % in pedestrians killed in road traffic accidents. Persons with blood alcohol levels of this order are clearly unable to look after themselves.

MEDICAL RECORDS

In any case of criminal violence the doctor who examines the victim will be asked to make a statement to the police. If a person is charged with an offence arising out of a physical assault the doctor may be required to give evidence in court and, if so, his original notes may be examined by both the prosecution and defence and the doctor may be examined and cross-examined upon these notes. It is, therefore, of major importance that the notes taken at the examination are complete and legible. On occasions it may be that the patient's condition is so critical that treatment is undertaken at once and so notes must be made later. It should be done as soon as possible. In practice, delays sometimes lead to major omissions which will be seized upon during the trial and will do nothing to enhance the doctor's reputation! In one case a second stab wound of the heart was not recorded after an emergency and unsuccessful thoracotomy to relieve tamponade. The defence was that this second stab wound was made accidentally by the thoracic surgeon! It must be remembered that even apparently trivial injuries may assume disproportionate importance in court.

When giving evidence in court a doctor may refer to his original notes and these may include laboratory tests, radiographs, etc. made during the course of treatment. In practice, one prepares a statement from one's notes and is usually asked about the origin of that report. It is essential that the original notes are taken to court as counsel may object to the report being used to 'refresh the memory'.

Many doctors have an aversion to appearing in court, usually because of a mistaken belief that their evidence will be pulled to pieces by counsel appearing for the other side. In practice this is not so, provided the doctor adheres to the facts and gives an honest opinion within the limits of his experience and expertise. More respect is accorded to the doctor who admits he does not know the answer than to the one who tries to give an opinion outside his specific field of knowledge.

Index